Psychiatry and the Humanities, Volume 6

Interpreting Lacan

Assistant Editor
Gloria H. Parloff

Editorial Assistant
Carolyn Wheaton

Editorial Aide
Katherine S. Henry

Published under the auspices of the
Forum on Psychiatry and the Humanities
The Washington School of Psychiatry

Psychiatry and the Humanities

VOLUME 6

Interpreting Lacan

Editors
Joseph H. Smith, M.D.
William Kerrigan, Ph.D.

New Haven and London   Yale University Press

Set in VIP Baskerville type by The Composing Room of
Michigan, Inc.
Printed in the United States of America by Vail-Ballou
Press, Binghamton, New York.

Library of Congress Cataloging in Publication Data

Main entry under title:

Interpreting Lacan.

(Psychiatry and the humanities; v. 6)
Includes index.
Contents: Introduction/by William Kerrigan—
Analysis. The image and the word/by Stanley A.
Leavy—Language, psychosis, and the subject in Lacan/
by John P. Muller—[etc.]
1. Psychoanalysis—Addresses, essays, lectures.
2. Lacan, Jacques, 1901–1981.—Addresses, essays,
lectures. I. Smith, Joseph H., 1927–   . II. Kerrigan,
William, 1943–   . III. Series.
RC321.P943 vol. 6   616.89s   83-7022
[RC509]   [616.89′17]
ISBN 0-300-03039-8

10   9   8   7   6   5   4   3   2   1

Contributors

Edward S. Casey, Ph.D. Professor of Philosophy and Chairman, Department of Philosophy, State University of New York at Stony Brook

André Green, M.D. Training Analyst, Paris Psychoanalytic Institute; formerly Chief, Clinic of Mental Diseases, Paris University

Julia Kristeva. Professor of Linguistics, University of Paris VII; Visiting Professor, Department of French, Columbia University; Psychoanalyst, Institute of Psychoanalysis, Paris

Stanley A. Leavy, M.D. Clinical Professor of Psychiatry, Yale University School of Medicine; Training and Supervising Analyst, Western New England Institute for Psychoanalysis

John P. Muller, Ph.D. Senior Researcher and member of the therapy staff, Austen Riggs Center, Stockbridge, Massachusetts

William J. Richardson, Ph.D. Professor of Philosophy, Boston College, and practicing psychoanalyst; formerly Director of Research, Austen Riggs Center, Stockbridge, Massachusetts

Christine van Boheemen-Saaf, Ph.D. Lecturer in English and American literature and literary theory, English Department, University of Leiden, The Netherlands

Wilfried Ver Eecke, Ph.D. Professor in Philosophy, and Chairman, Department of Philosophy, Georgetown University, Washington, D.C.

Antoine Vergote, Phil. D. Professor of Psychology and Philosophy, Katholieke Universiteit Leuven-Belgium; President of the Ecole Belge de Psychanalyse

J. Melvin Woody, Ph.D. Professor of Philosophy, Connecticut College, New London

Contents

Introduction

WILLIAM KERRIGAN

Jacques Lacan was born in 1901—seven years after Heinz Hartmann, three years after Rudolph Loewenstein, one year after Ernst Kris, one year before Erik Erikson, and a decade before David Rapaport. He belonged, in other words, to the generation of psychoanalytic theorists who were able to imagine that Freud, a living presence for about half their lives, might really have been their father—and the French son was intensely aware of his position with respect to his imaginative siblings. To his mind there was scant difference among the others but a substantial gap between them and himself. As he needed to remind us over and over again in his shameless and obstreperous way, he was in his own view the hardest one to like—a self-image that did not, however, prompt him to deny himself the pleasures of sniping at the fame and institutional security of the others. No chocolates, flowers, and smiles in his courtship of renown, but rather unwelcome truths set down in a knowingly obscure style. Where the others (in his view) sought to complete a psychology of the individual with a sociology of functional adaptation, Lacan looked toward an anthropology grounded on bare schemata; where they would sweeten the vulgar tongue of the id with the humanist wisdom of literature, Lacan turned to the harrowing abstractions of linguistics and mathematics; where they explored the cognitive autonomy and intrasystemic harmonies of the ego, Lacan indicted its every pretense to majesty. Lacan to Lacan was the *difficult* one whose hard lessons would preserve for our continued meditation what the tranquilizing thoughts of his peers would cover over: Freud. His was not a Freud you could go beyond, because his meaning had no distinct boundary. Lacan was attuned to those moments in the writings of Freud that lie between the fixities of evidence and theory, moments of puzzlement or intellectual trauma when, in the face of disbelief, psychoanalysis is arising.

He wanted to recover nothing more and nothing less than the roots of it: the living Freud, not the answerer exhibited in handbooks and paraphrases. Lacan's repeated claim to inhabit the living meaning of Sigmund Freud cannot be dismissed as readily as some suppose. Whatever else we may wish to say about his work, it should be granted at the outset that Lacan was indeed an extraordinary exegete. Today, in the burgeoning field of hermeneutics, philosopher-critics debate whether meaning is stable and selfsame or rather changes along with interpreters and their circumstances. The common objection to the second position is that it offers no warrant for correcting someone who has read carelessly or come away from a text with an obviously impoverished or wrongheaded account of its purport. But as Harold Bloom implies in his emphasis on the "strong" misreading, there are no consequential philosophical problems in maintaining that, once again and in familiar ways, Doctor A, Professor B, or media person C has "misread" Freud. Something altogether different happens when Lacan, who if a misreader is surely a strong one, discovers the mind of Freud groping intuitively in instance upon instance for a scientific linguistics that it does not possess. Only the unorthodox *and* impressive reading meaningfully agitates the doctrine of stable sense. As with Plotinus on Plato and Ficino on Plotinus, so with Lacan on Freud: in order to address the question of whether an author has been distorted, we must first rethink, in terms the exegete has provided us with, the essential problems posed in the texts of this author. The many psychoanalytic essays that begin by reviewing the literature, including Freud, then proceed to supplement and correct this body of past discourse, teach us little or nothing about what Freud meant. Those who claim to go beyond Freud teach us little or nothing about what Freud meant. Like no one else in his generation, Lacan has the power to throw us back with new urgency to the texts—the power to disturb and reinitiate our sense of Freud.

Lacan died as we were preparing this book in 1981, at the age of eighty. The age revealed in the obituaries surprised a lot of people. Could someone of such recent fame be so old? The tardy assimilation of Lacan into our language is an interesting tale and, for understanding his current place in English-speaking psychoanalysis, a necessary one.

The *stade du miroir*—the earliest idea, both psychogenetically and in the career of Lacan's thought—was formulated in the 1930s. But it was in the 1950s, after the hiatus of World War II, that Lacan enjoyed his most creative period; all of the great papers on language in *Écrits* date from this time. In 1953, when the split in the Société Psychanalytique de Paris occasioned the first of these statements, "Fonction et champ de la parole et du langage en psychanalyse" (sometimes known as the "Discours de Rome"), Lacan also published his first essay in English, "Some Reflections on the Ego," which appeared—with an irony that would not have escaped the author—in the *International Journal of Psycho-Analysis,* the organ of the association that would that very year deny legitimacy to the group led by Lacan and Daniel Lagache. Delivered before the British Psychoanalytic Society in 1951, "Some Reflections on the Ego" contains a summary of the theory of the mirror phase, a brief account of the relationship between metaphor and hysterical conversion, and some characteristic vituperation on the ego as a fatally narcissistic structure. But as Wilden has said, this paper "does not come over with the verve and thought-provoking virtuosity one expects from Lacan" (1966, p. 263). His second English publication, written with Wladimir Franoff, appears in *Perversions: Psychodynamics and Therapy* (1956), a volume of essays edited by Sandor Lorand and Michael Balint. It is now an odd experience to read through this collection of worthy if uninspired work and, near the end of the book, come upon Lacan's "Fetishism: The Symbolic, the Imaginary and the Real." For there he is, fully himself, laconic and lacunary, evoking as he often does the epigrammatic, grandly definitive manner of the Pre-Socratics while dividing all of psychoanalysis into the now-famous three parts:

> And if we consider mankind's first words, we note that the password, for instance, has the function—as a sign of recognition— of saving its speaker from death.
> The word is a gift of language and language is not imma-

terial. It is subtle matter, but matter nonetheless. It can fe-
cundate the hysterical woman, it can stand for the flow of
urine or for excrement withheld. Words can also suffer symbolic wounds. We recall the "Wespe" with a castrated W,
when the wolf man realized the symbolic punishment which
was inflicted upon him by Grouscha.

Language is thus the symbolic activity *par excellence;* all
theories of language based on a confusion between the word
and its referent overlook this essential dimension. Does not
Humpty Dumpty remind Alice that he is master of the word,
if not of its referent?

The imaginary is decipherable only if it is rendered into
symbols. [p. 269]

In fetishism the three domains are arrayed with particular clarity.
The Real (the absence of the maternal phallus), unable to be
registered in the Symbolic (entered into language and experienced as true), will yield to the Imaginary (the fetish). The genesis
of the fetish is, moreover, a parable for the partial, truncated
relationship of the unconscious to the Symbolic that the analyst,
through his deciphering interpretations, attempts to complete.
Here as elsewhere Lacan insists on the primacy of the signifier:
"language is not immaterial." Gratuitous and wholly alogical like-
nesses of sound and orthography supply a network into which the
id spreads in dreams, jokes, parapraxias, and free associations. In
this matrix of linguistic *materia,* which Lacan calls the "essential
dimension," the unconscious speaks, repudiating from within
symbolic activity itself the false autonomy of the speaking ego.
Words in the primary process are treated *as images,* and in this
sense we may say that for Lacan the fundamental discovery of
psychoanalysis, the unconscious, is in effect a universal and involuntary fetishism of the signifier.

Nobody listened in 1956. A weird little paper on fetishism, at
least ostensibly: so what else is new? During the next decade,
when the writings and seminars of Lacan disseminated his influence throughout French culture, he was virtually unknown in
England and America; the maverick thinker who troubled En-

glish-speaking psychoanalysis at this time (the one you were sure to be asked about, the one on whom, in order to be au courant, you had to ready a judgment in three or four pithy sentences, to be uttered only after a pause simulating genuine reflection) was R. D. Laing, not Jacques Lacan. The first essay in English devoted to the work of Lacan came in 1966, and its author, Anthony Wilden, was not a psychoanalyst but a graduate student studying Montaigne. Lacan—and this is one reason he is an appropriate subject for the present series of volumes—came into our language largely through the conduit of the humanities; Wilden's essay was, in fact, published in *American Imago*. Also in 1966, *Yale French Studies* brought out its famous double issue on structuralism, containing the first translation of Lacan for a decade and, again by Wilden, an annotated bibliography of his works. Still, for yet another decade Lacan was more read about than read. It was not until 1977, when Sheridan's selected translation of *Écrits* appeared in England, that enough of Lacan existed in our language to permit a serious encounter.

The analytic community is not entirely to blame for this unfortunate neglect: leaders failed. In 1971 Heinz Kohut displaced R. D. Laing as the-one-who-must-be-classified-quickly with the publication of *The Analysis of the Self*, which is importantly concerned with narcissistic "mirroring" and the "mirror transference" of the borderline patient. Almost unbelievably, though for thirty years Lacan's work had borne on such matters, he is not mentioned. (He *is* mentioned in *The Restoration of the Self*, Kohut's 1977 sequel to his first book—on a list with nine other theorists whom, despite admitted overlapping with his own thought, Kohut will not discuss.) When Kernberg appeared on the heels of Kohut, leading some people in the profession of psychotherapy to behave as if the regnant issue of their historical moment were the choice between the one or the other, or the achievement of some satisfactory combination of the two, the advice to the intellectually curious had not improved—no mention of Lacan in the papers gathered in Kernberg's *Borderline Conditions and Pathological Narcissism* (1975). So it was that while humanists such as Eugen Bär and Fredric Jameson were treating Lacan as the major psychoanalytic theorist of his generation, the leading theorists of English-speaking psychoanalysis proceeded in apparent ignorance of his work, even when the questions at issue were congruent with those of Lacan. Schafer does not allude to Lacan in *A New Language for Psychoanalysis* (1976), nor does Loewald in his *Papers on Psychoanalysis* (1980). In his *Language and Interpretation in Psychoanalysis* (1975), Edelson is happily aware that "one might well ask why in a book on psychoanalysis and language there is no use made of the work of Jacques Lacan" (p. 7), and answers in a passage bristling with a fatigued author's grouchy unwillingness to absorb another major influence that Lacan is "prophetic and evangelical (I distrust charisma)," holds a view of language unenlightened by Chomsky, is philosophical in the continental way (phenomenology and existentialism), sets great store in drafty words such as "other," and "is on the whole not my cup of tea" (p. 10). To my knowledge, this was the first extended comment on Lacan by an American psychoanalyst.

Finally the boom began: an issue of *Yale French Studies* given over to the "French Freud" (1976); the translation of Anika Lemaire's *Jacques Lacan* (1977), with a thoughtful preface by Antoine Vergote; Sheridan's translation of some of the seminars, *The Four Fundamental Concepts of Psycho-Analysis* (1978), as a companion volume to his *Écrits*; Ver Eecke's translation of De Waelhens' *Schizophrenia* (1978); two books dealing primarily with the therapeutic dimension of Lacan's work, Leavy's *The Psychoanalytic Dialogue* (1980) and Schneiderman's anthology *Returning to Freud: Clinical Psychoanalysis in the School of Lacan* (1980); and the articles of Muller and Richardson in *Psychoanalysis and Contemporary Thought* (now collected in *Lacan and Language: A Reader's Guide to Écrits*). Suddenly Lacan was the darling of English psychoanalytic chatter. What about *him*? And then he was dead.

A major irony of this story lies in the fact that the most thoughtful arguments against Lacan's renovation of psychoanalysis were available in English before Lacan's own works. In *Freud and Philosophy* (1970), probably the finest contribution to psychoanalysis by a nonanalyst, Paul Ricoeur presupposes Lacan from the beginning—indeed, especially from the beginning. The book opens with a dramatic expansion of Lacan's various assaults on the *cogito* of Descartes and Husserl, setting the unconscious, which can only be discovered through a labor of interpretation, against the self-evident consciousness of the phenomenology in which Ricoeur was trained. Then, after situating psychoanalysis in a general theory of symbolism, Ricoeur commences interpreting Freud with a defense of psychic energy as a concept poised between biology and semantics, reducible to neither. Many readers have been puzzled or put off by this slow, laboriously detailed account of Freudian energics. It may help to realize that what is really at stake in this section of *Freud and Philosophy* is Lacan: Ricoeur is interpreting the underpinnings of psychoanalysis in such a way that, much later in the argument (pp. 395–415), Lacan's linguistic unconscious can be discarded as an untenable distortion—a movement from the biological determinism Freud sometimes espoused to a new structuralist determinism of the "not immaterial" signifier. As Ricoeur maintained more explicitly in a subsequent essay, the linguistic unconscious renders phenomena closely associated with psychic energy in Freud's thought, such as resistance, incomprehensible (1981, pp. 257–58). In his encyclopedic work *The Rule of Metaphor,* published in the same year as Sheridan's translations of Lacan, Ricoeur continued his long intellectual battle against the explanatory tyranny of enclosed and self-referential structures by presenting good metaphor as both an advent of a novel meaning unpredictable on the basis of a semantics of synchronic order, in which the meaning of any one term consists in its differential relationship to all the terms, and at the same time as fully referential, an invitation to redescribe the world. These issues reappear in the volume at hand. Where, in all this talk about signifiers, is the world—the ultimate sense of the signified? If our advancing knowledge of language is to enrich Freudian thought, what are the psychic analogues to good metaphor? Although Lacan is at last available to us in English, questions like these may make him appear to be already behind us. The best minds have agreed upon his failings; alternatives have been proposed; feminists have found in him yet another psychoanalytic villain. Why not pass on to other subjects?

Because it is important right now not to chatter about Lacan, not to dismiss him with a few sentences, not to allow a list of his shortcomings, however accurate, to substitute for a serious engagement with his work. For the work is spacious—and difficult. To assimilate a writer so allusive as Lacan is to enter into an entire culture. English-speaking psychoanalysis has tended to conceive of itself in the piecemeal fashion encouraged by empirical science. Is this item of Freudian doctrine correct? By what sort of study could we demonstrate its reliability? These are worthy concerns, but there should be room as well for another way of working through Freud's achievement. However firm his grounding in Freud, the reader of Lacan will be likely to find himself, in ways that may initially be quite uncomfortable, a student; he must learn to think psychoanalysis with a speculative breadth sometimes exceeding that of Freud himself. Evidence comes from all quarters of the humanities, and it comes quickly, without the guidance of a transition: Lacan delights in brief but intense episodes of erudition. Richard Rorty, in a charming essay (1980) that diagnoses and attempts to cure a certain skittish defensiveness in psychoanalytic discourse, has suggested that the healthiest thing we might do about Freud at this moment in our history is simply to let him sink in. Like victims of a blow, we know that something authoritative has been done to us, but, still reeling, we have yet to assess the damage—or perhaps the improvement, since that blow might have prevented us from continuing on a dangerous, or hopeless, course. This is good advice, with Lacan as with Freud. The truly fertile critiques of Lacan will come from those who, tossed in the churn of his texts, have been permanently changed by him.

This book is designed to ease its reader into the process of interpreting Lacan. It begins with three essays centered on the application of his thought to the work of therapy. Stanley Leavy offers a broad introduction to Lacanianism for American psychoanalysts, and by pointing to the dominance of speech in the therapeutic situation makes a general case for the plausibility of a thoroughgoing linguistic transformation of Freud. John Muller, noting the congruence between the *stade du miroir* and contemporary developments in cognitive psychology, ends with a concrete instance of how the Lacanian version of the "talking cure" functioned in the treatment of a schizophrenic patient. After restating in linguistic terms Freud's distinction between primary and secondary process, Julia Kristeva focuses on the analyst's response to the "empty" speech of a borderline patient. As the reader proceeds to the second, longest and most demanding section of this volume, on the philosophical elements in Lacan, he or she should bear in mind Kristeva's intriguing remarks about the kind and timing of interpretive intervention in the borderline discourse, for she provides a rejoinder of sorts to the criticisms of Lacanian therapy voiced at the end of this section by Antoine Vergote.

In the first of the philosophical essays William Richardson concentrates on the beheaded "subject" that Lacan raises like a Medusa's head before the well-armed ego of American and British psychoanalysis. If Lacan would prefer to say, not that the unconscious lives us, but that the unconscious speaks us, the implications remain the same—an unbending determinism and a systematic inversion of Cartesian themes, such that the subject becomes effect rather than cause, structured rather than structuring, and doubtful in its certainty rather than certain in its doubtfulness. Lacan turns away from the ancient question of the unity of the subject; his guiding orientation, which Richardson brings to light in recounting Lacan's attack on Erikson's interpretation of the Irma dream, is disorientation—rupture, split, decomposition. The key to the famous dream, and to the unconscious itself, resides in a chemical formula, a reading very much in line with Lacan's own increasing preoccupation with mathematical formalism. But would it be possible, Richardson concludes, to think the unity of the subject in a manner answerable to Lacanian themes? He suggests that this project would involve, contrary to Lacan's own movement toward mathematical models, a reaffirmation of the Hegelian and Heideggerian elements in his work.

It is to just these aspects of Lacan that the next three chapters are addressed. Edward Casey and J. Melvin Woody argue that Lacan, by deploying Hegelian desire (a desire that becomes "human" in being aimed at what is human in the other: his desire) and such Heideggerian notions as the temporal "ecstasies" (also unique to the *Dasein* of human being), liberates psychoanalysis from the "reduction" to physicalistic, therefore quantifiable, and therefore subhuman drives in Freud. This suspicion of the economic point of view is by now so traditional in philosophical responses to Freud that one tends not to notice: contemporary psychoanalysis, within the circumscription of its own literature, is well aware of the problem. But the reader should pay close attention to the polemic against Ricoeur in this essay, for as previously indicated, the great originality of Ricoeur among philosophical commentators on Freud lies in his lengthy appreciation for the wisdom of the founder's economics. We often find that we do not know how to value something until we have been deprived of it, and one of the interesting consequences of Lacan's linguistics of the unconscious is to show us what a complexly elaborated psychoanalysis looks like without the baseline of energics. This matter resurfaces in the papers of Green and Vergote.

Wilfried Ver Eecke covers much the same ground as that half of the Casey-Woody essay devoted to Hegel, but he emphasizes that the theory of the mirror phase is not Hegelian merely: Lacan makes himself responsible to facts about animals, accepting the biological context that Casey and Woody find inherently reductive in the work of Freud. Indeed, the theory of the mirror phase runs together two kinds of necessity, that of presumed scientific fact and that of dialectical logic—and the second of these appears less "necessary" the more one examines the difference between Lacan's projection of ego genesis and Hegel's logical explication of the rivalry between self-consciousnesses. Might the mirror phase be conceived of as a speculative prehistory of the Hegelian encounter? This question assumes that a philosophical reading of Lacan, determined to think through with all due rigor the "unsaid" in his frequent allusions to philosophy, would be both appropriate and fruitful. Might it not be better, as Ver Eecke implies, to abandon this enterprise, concluding instead that philosophical ideas served Lacan as metaphors and indicators, ways of pointing toward his insights rather than constituting them?

Richardson strenuously rejects this option in his second contribution. His large effort here is to open out the philosophical and theological horizons that Lacan himself, like Freud before him, endeavored to shut down. There is some warrant for doing so, even at the heart of Lacan's work; one might detect the rudiments of something like a Christian psycho-theology in his master trope for subjectivity: the wound. But Richardson does not go so far as this. Drawing on his double expertise in philosophy and psychoanalysis, he attempts to position Lacanian subjectivity in the kinetic disclosure of the "Being-question." We can say of Lacan's unconscious that it cannot be mastered by conscious volition or by metaphysical concept; that it can after a fashion be affirmed, as in the psychoanalytic treatment; that it belongs intrinsically to the way in which language is given to our species, and puts us in touch with some of the primordial functions of language, as when in free association it lays out signifiers side by side; that it is, by constantly recombining its elements, constantly revealing itself, if only in the form of error; that a withdrawal or concealment belongs essentially to the mode of its revealing; and that this concealment is itself regularly concealed from us. Parallel statements emerge in Heidegger's late explorations of Being. As with Being, so with Lacan's linguistic unconscious: if we acknowledge that structural linguistics can handle no more than what is revealed, there remains in the process of our existence a mystery known only in our recognition of its concealment. It is Richardson's bet that this convergence supplies the new psychoanalysis of Lacan with a grounding in human existence.

André Green's essay will probably require several readings. It is the most esoteric piece in this collection, an example of High Lacanianism composed when Green was attending Lacan's seminar and caught up in the excitement of his teaching. The reader's patience may not survive a first try: really now, what does the metaphysics of zero have to do with psychoanalysis? The author informs us in an introduction written for this appearance of his essay, the first in English, that he himself has abandoned such high jinks for the clearer and clinically oriented teachings of Winnicott and Bion. But we make no apologies for this contribution. Green notes important failings in Lacan, contrasts him with

Freud in a way that illuminates both figures, offers a theory integrating anxiety as "signal" or "signifier" with the linguistic unconscious, finding time along the way for a telling observation about *Hamlet,* a brilliant interpretation of the handkerchief in *Othello,* and a rich suggestion about how Judaic themes resonate in Freud's late concern with anxiety (the iconoclastic sign, the sign unaccompanied by representation) and the death drive (the "silence" that walls off the subject of the afterlife)—and all this while explicating several of Lacan's diagrams!

Whereas other contributors have focused on the subject in Lacan, Green turns to the object, specifically to the notion of the *objet a.*[1] A few remarks about this concept may aid the interested reader. The *objet a* is Lacan's name for the various transformations "want" or "lack" or "not being" undergoes in psychic development. Previous essays have considered the first appearance (inseparably the first concealment) of this unbearably real privation, when it is covered over in the jubilation of the mirror phase. Green retraces the full genealogy of this "want." Identified with the maternal phallus, eventual successor to the maternal gestalt, the ego is once again in the image of an ideal and of what is not. We are still in the realm of the Imaginary: the ego will discover this "want" in the mother and in itself in a visual mode. At this point a precise phenomenology leads Green into the peculiarities of zero. For lack *is not seen*; vision, strictly speaking, can behold only what is there. In the unconscious this unrepresentable lack generates chains of signifiers representing either the vagina or its denial, but both chains proceed from the imageless lack; at the core of this structure is the death drive, that dispersal or noniden-

1. The full term in Lacan is usually *objet petit a,* where the "little 'a'" in question derives from *autre* (other). Although Alan Sheridan complied with Lacan's wish that *objet petit a* "should remain untranslated, thus acquiring, as it were, the status of an algebraic sign" (*Écrits,* p. xi), there are already signs of slippage. We have chosen to keep the conception French, since strict translations such as "object o" may give the mistaken impression that the "o" has been detached from "object" instead of "other." However, following the lead of French commentators, we permit ourselves to elide the *petit.* In contexts where confusion might result, such as in André Green's essay in this volume, *objet a* also appears as *objet (a).*

tity that has no signifier. So the absence of the maternal phallus is the "want" in psychogenesis analogous to the zero in mathematics—the generative number, nonidentical with itself, that the other numbers, identical with themselves, both require and cancel. Green sees in the *objet a* an escape from the oppressive binarism of structuralist thought. From the "want" issue two chains of signifiers, differing from each other as plus to minus, but the "want," the center of a binary structure that is not itself captured within the structure, belongs to neither. Possessing a maturational gradient as well, the lack that cannot be seen evokes *knowledge,* and at the end of a positive oedipal settlement, "want" in this sense will have positioned the ego in the social realm of law and language. Green's essay, then, is a meditation on the trauma dividing the mirror phase (the Imaginary) from the Name-of-the-Father (the Symbolic). It is evident from his conclusion that we have not, for all the pyrotechnics here, broken free from the pervasive Lacanian desire to scourge narcissistic forms of subjectivity.

Green seems divided between two responses to Lacan—to use Freud in order to strengthen and solidify the new paradigms of Lacan, or to use the sturdiest innovations of Lacan to strengthen and solidify the original paradigms of Freud. Casey and Woody, Richardson, and to some extent Ver Eecke follow the first path: Lacan is now the preferable model, the place where Freud has been relocated. In the last of our theoretical essays, Vergote takes the second path. The linguistic unconscious cannot account for affect or resistance. In his lopsided dedication to the signifier, Lacan mounts a theory that is impotent before the great issues of meaning and reference; he leaves us not in the world but in a closed circuit of signifiers. More specifically, his failure to resume the Freudian theme of the "thing-presentation," and thus to allow for some sort of differentiation between a signifier and a signified, results in the empty speech of a schizophrenic unconscious. Our subjective life is more anchored, more unified, and more deeply enmeshed with the otherness of the signified than Lacan assumes. It is hoped that Vergote's essay will also lend a certain unity to the reader's experience of this volume. By deducing from Lacan's theoretical positions the insufficiencies of a therapy derived from them, Vergote casts us back with new questions to the more modest clinical chapters with which the book begins.

No interpretation is complete, Heidegger maintained, giving his own stamp to a venerable idea implicit in Western hermeneutics from Plato's quest for the beautiful to Freud's conception of the psychoanalytic cure, without an "event of appropriation." In the spirit of this tradition we close with a single example of using Lacan—Christine van Boheemen-Saaf's essay on *Bleak House*. Poets and novelists seem always to be anticipating psychoanalysts. Certainly the dark world encroaching on Esther Summerson gives concrete form to the issues that interpreting Lacan expose for us. Law has deteriorated into automatic writing: origins have slipped away, fogbound, threatening us with the vision of a universal orphanhood. Questions debated elsewhere in this book in philosophical and linguistic terms coalesce here about the extended index finger of Inspector Bucket, which directs Esther back to the securities of a fixed identity. Does the psychoanalysis of Lacan underwrite the fulfillment of this sign? Or does it rather, by detaching this sign from the anchorage of the world, abandon us to a "want" filled only by the restless permutations of a mad language?

Whatever our answer, we are not done with interpreting Lacan, for he is not the sort of author who can be made obsolete by the detection of serious flaws in his thinking. To appreciate the antisystematic vitality of this writer it is crucial to realize that he was, in truth, a man of words: no psychoanalyst has ever mastered, or sought to master, such a style. This is not to say, of course, that Freud was a middling stylist. He wrote with grace and wit, and in his best moments put us in touch with something unique—a peculiar human dignity that, while commanding tragic power, remained uninflated, disciplined to allow itself no more than the just degree of pride. But the greatness of this rhetorical achievement can be measured by our unawareness of it. For long stretches we see only the subject matter, the progress of the argument; our subliminal sense of Freud's trustworthiness results to some extent from his humble willingness to (seemingly) efface his presence. We feel that he wants only to convince us in the noblest way, without rhetorical guile, and not to entangle us in any costly fashion with himself as the dispenser of our wisdom.

But Lacan, although a great exegete, did not adopt the transparency of style conventionally associated with exegetical commentary. If Freud is Homer or Sophocles, Lacan is Nonnos or Seneca: rhetoric has claimed a world unto itself through which we must pass, meeting demands, if we would know what the author knows. Freud was at his greatest as a writer when confronting the theme of fate, which is, in all its ramifications, the fundamental subject of his psychoanalysis. Lacan, however, tells his seminar (as quoted by Richardson on p. 63): "The game is already played, the dice are already cast. . . . Don't you find something ridiculous and laughable in the fact that the dice are [already] cast?" This is far from the quiet solemnity, the attempt to strike some kind of psychic equilibrium before *Ananke,* that we find in Freud. In Lacan's thought the concept of *jouissance,* the pleasure that does not end in equilibration, embodies this amusement in the face of the preordained. Translated into a style, *jouissance* plays everywhere in the discourse of this psychoanalyst.

It is somehow perfectly right that the first English champion of Lacan should have been a student of Montaigne, for in his seminars particularly, Lacan often reminds us of the man who invented the essay (*Essais, Écrits*) as a genre for declaring selfhood:

> Well . . . Freud tells us repeatedly that sublimation is also satisfaction of the drive, whereas it is *zielgehemmt,* inhibited as to its aim—it does not attain it. Sublimation is nonetheless satisfaction of the drive, without repression.
>
> In other words—for the moment, I am not fucking, I am talking to you. Well! I can have exactly the same satisfaction as if I were fucking. That's what it means. Indeed, it raises the question of whether in fact I am not fucking at this moment. [1978, pp. 165–66]

A witty exposure of paradoxes inherent in Freud's idea of sublimation? Yes, but we might also be listening to a modernist variation on Montaigne's famous "Quand je dance, je dance; quand je dors, je dors," the spirit of which one modern scholar has attempted to render in "When I dance, I dance; when I fuck, I fuck" (Quinones, 1972, p. 242); it is pleasant to imagine that the greatest French narcissist, as a fellow sufferer of the sweet symptoms of logophilia, would have assented to this condensation of the intensities of experience he himself had been proud of separating. Writing a speech for the unconscious, Lacan has this "Freudian thing" tell us that it speaks in "the most farfetched conceit" (*la pointe la plus gongorique*)" (1977, p. 122), an allusion to the seventeenth-century aesthetic of Gongorism, whose English incarnation was in the so-called metaphysical poets. It is in this sort of style that Lacan has chosen to clothe himself. His language is taut with intellect, but an intellect compelled to display itself, even turn against itself, in irrational excesses—hyperbole, indirection, percussive juxtaposition, a whole array of stylistic disinhibitions aiming to produce, not an invisible marriage of thought and language, but the *impression* thought makes on the "not immaterial" substance of language. "Indeed, it raises the question of whether in fact I am not fucking at this moment."

Lacan, Malcolm Bowie has noted (1979, pp. 143–49, 151–52), deliberately frustrates our desire to receive from psychoanalytic discourse a firm conceptual model able to be attacked or affirmed, paraphrased or applied. To be sure, he does not lack for conceptual models. They are plentiful, and like rabbits from a hat, mysterious by their proliferation. Often discarded as soon as they are built, the models are built strangely—from the roof downward, or resting in midair, with glass walls and plaster windows. We find in his prose all of the paraphernalia of *clarté*. But it is the clarity of Magritte. Lacan is rife with theorems, technical neologisms, formulas, graphs, exposures of competing positions. Yet the theorems tend to explode outward into other branches of knowledge rather than to tighten the internal structure of his psychoanalysis; the formulas and the graphs do not so much summarize his exposition as replace it, permitting Lacan to meander off into the implications and consequences of an argument he has really yet to fix; the polemics against competitors appear, not when the argument dictates, but apparently whenever Lacan feels like it, which is often. In this opponent of the *cogito,* the stylistic gestures of Cartesian *clarté* are made to serve a wavering and multiplicate meaning. Lacan, to put this another way, was a deeply intuitive thinker who was drawn to appropriating and fracturing a set of stylistic conventions forged primarily by those who thought at the opposite pole of the intellectual world.

Throughout the history of literature—in the wrathful rant of Senecan tragedy, the drunken epic of Nonnos, the rapturous self-scrutiny of Montaigne, the torn arcadia of Góngora—such conflictual rhetoric is found in close proximity to a drastic and therefore potentially elusive or problematic selfhood. These are texts that force critics to make an other than programmatic distinction between author and persona. Lacan, like the surrealists whom he admired, reanimates this distinction in a Freudian setting. The subject must speak, and for Lacan the subject is an unconscious author, the ego mere persona. As a writer, then, Lacan attempts to make sense while also allowing a "nonsense sense," the energy of the unconscious, to run through his signifiers—hence, for example, the prevalence of the pun. We know that signifiers are arbitrary; there is no logical explanation for the line of poetry in "universe" or the philosopher in "likewise." But in punning these alogical connections are made to seem necessary and truth-bearing, and for the punster who enters the sphere of the ego from a realm of unmeaning, these whims of the signifier give expression to psychic life in its most primordial form (*lettre/l'être*). Lacan seeks by intellectual means to let *it* speak. The crisscrossing of signifiers in his texts may supply another reason, different from the one assumed in this volume's philosophical essays, for those odd appeals to Heidegger whenever the subject of the cure emerges. Though he lacks the tone of somber reverence that informs even the polemics in Heidegger, Lacan's thought, like Heidegger's, is hung on a spreading concatenation of signifiers: *Holzwege* that led Heidegger through the forgotten forests of Being, and if Lacan is right, led Freud to the very locus of the forgotten.

Even should his stature in psychoanalysis prove inconsiderable once all the chatter has died away, Lacan may well be found among the few psychoanalysts to have earned a place in the memory of the humanities.

REFERENCES

Bowie, M. "Jacques Lacan." In J. Sturrock, ed., *Structuralism and Since: From Lévi-Strauss to Derrida*. Oxford: Oxford University Press, 1979.

De Waelhens, A. *Schizophrenia*. Translated by W. Ver Eecke. Pittsburgh: Duquesne University Press, 1978.

Edelson, M. *Language and Interpretation in Psychoanalysis*. New Haven: Yale University Press, 1975.

Kernberg, O. *Borderline Conditions and Pathological Narcissism*. New York: Jason Aronson, 1975.

Kohut, H. *The Analysis of the Self*. New York: International Universities Press, 1971.

———. *The Restoration of the Self*. New York: International Universities Press, 1977.

Lacan, J. "Some Reflections on the Ego." *International Journal of Psycho-Analysis* 34 (1953): 11–17.

———. "Fetishism: The Symbolic, the Imaginary and the Real." In S. Lorand and M. Balint, eds., *Perversions: Psychodynamics and Therapy*. New York: Gramercy, 1956.

———. *Écrits: A Selection*. Translated by A. Sheridan. New York: Norton, 1977.

———. *The Four Fundamental Concepts of Psycho-Analysis*. Translated by A. Sheridan. New York: Norton, 1978.

Leavy, S. *The Psychoanalytic Dialogue*. New Haven: Yale University Press, 1980.

Lemaire, A. *Jacques Lacan*. Translated by D. Macey. London: Routledge, 1977.

Loewald, H. *Papers on Psychoanalysis*. New Haven: Yale University Press, 1980.

Muller, J. P., and Richardson, W. J. *Lacan and Language: A Reader's Guide to Écrits*. New York: International Universities Press, 1982.

Quinones, R. *The Renaissance Discovery of Time*. Cambridge, Mass.: Harvard University Press, 1972.

Ricoeur, P. *Freud and Philosophy*. Translated by D. Savage. New Haven: Yale University Press, 1970.

_____. *The Rule of Metaphor*. Translated by R. Czerny. Toronto: University of Toronto Press, 1977.

_____. *Hermeneutics and the Human Sciences*. Edited and translated by J. B. Thompson. Cambridge: Cambridge University Press, 1981.

Rorty, R. "Freud, Morality, and Hermeneutics." *New Literary History* 12 (1980): 177–86.

Schafer, R. *A New Language for Psychoanalysis*. New Haven: Yale University Press, 1976.

Schneiderman, S. *Returning to Freud: Clinical Psychoanalysis in the School of Lacan*. New Haven: Yale University Press, 1980.

Wilden, A. "Freud, Signorelli and Lacan: The Repression of the Signifier." *American Imago* 23 (1966): 332–77.

_____. "Jacques Lacan: A Partial Bibliography." *Yale French Studies* 36–37 (1966): 263–68.

Analysis

1

The Image and the Word: Further Reflections on Jacques Lacan

STANLEY A. LEAVY

> The mirror would do well to reflect a little more before returning our image to us.—Jacques Lacan (1977, p. 138)

In my earlier brief study of Jacques Lacan (1978), I presented, in an admittedly simplified form, my impressions of the "significance" of this radical thinker. I devoted most of my attention to his debt to the linguistic theories of Saussure and Jakobson and to the importance of his break with traditional psychoanalytic metapsychology. He seemed to me to be a substantial innovator, really the most important innovator since Freud. Until Lacan, innovation in psychoanalytic theory consisted either of extensions of Freud's manifest meaning or of approximations to social science or biology—Melanie Klein at one extreme, Heinz Hartmann at the other, one's preference depending on the appeal of an id psychology or an ego psychology. In either case, for all the fury of the dispute between the two, there was no basic departure from the theory of the structure and dynamics of the psyche as it appears in Freud's later writings.

The sociological movement might be illustrated by Erich Fromm, for whom a sometimes veiled social moralism governed theoretical conceptions, or by Erik Erikson, a far more profound thinker, but also one whose earlier allegiance to social science discouraged attention to the depths that Freud had first exposed. Of the biological side I will only say that it has tried to undo psychoanalysis by returning to Freud—before he was the Freud who made all the difference, when he located the "laboratory" of psychoanalysis in the consulting room.

3

Lacan's theoretical contributions are more radical than any of these movements because they strike at the center of the psychoanalytic situation itself. For Lacan it is the intersubjective position of psychoanalysis that is to be understood theoretically, not just the dynamics of the personality. Whence such aphorisms as "the transference is the desire of the analyst," a statement that needs to be taken in its full ambiguity and that rests on two conceptions: the subject as an image derived from other subjects and the communication through language of the otherness of the subject. It is not that these and many other ideas are opposed to Freudian formulations, any more than that they are merely translations of well-known principles into a strange vocabulary. Both contentions have been made against Lacan, but they miss the point: Lacan has been trying to rebuild psychoanalysis from the ground up, the ground being the language, or more properly, the speaking in which the analysis takes place. He does not operate without presuppositions, but his are different presuppositions from Freud's. For all Lacan's early training as physician and psychiatrist, he does not think of patients as persons "having" neuroses, the causes for which need to be investigated by means of analysis so that a redistribution of energies can take place. For Lacan symptoms are themselves metaphors, even when they are spoken by the body, and the analysis is really analysis of language, the therapeutic aim being the discovery by speaking of what it is whereof the patient speaks. I hope that I shall at least indirectly make some of this a little plainer in the course of this essay. For Lacan is far from plain.

It was only right that the *enfant terrible* of psychoanalysis should be a Frenchman. It is not merely a question of national character, always a debatable explanation, although a tempting one for the foreigner—the unique complex of dramatic display, preciosity of expression, the *succès de scandale,* pitched battles between rival intellectual camps, taken together with the mordant wit we call Gallic. None of this accounts for the appearance of a Jacques Lacan on the French scene. Of more serious moment might be the fact that until he appeared, French psychoanalysis looked like not much more than a translation of the Germanic and Anglo-

American schools. There have been some exceptions, but no matter; before the challenge of Lacan, French psychoanalysis was hardly an indispensable resource, and worse still, it was not of much influence in France. That has all changed, and the changes are by no means to be found only within the number of those who have had the pontifical approval of Lacan.[1]

Another matter that deserves comment is Lacan's disposition to ridicule. It is not the way I would go about at length trying to advance psychoanalysis, and incontestably, it has frequently been wounding and even destructive. But psychoanalysis—whether more than other sciences I do not know—has been disposed to nurture sacred cows, eminences whose every innocent rumination has been taken as something like Holy Writ. This has struck me as suspiciously like the effects of the transference that it is our business to resolve (plus expertness in public relations), and it has sometimes brought about an enforced and uncriticized domination under which new thinking has withered. Again, it is only human nature, if I may be naive, that Lacan became in time one of the most conspicuous of sacred cows himself, and at last, by a supreme irony, knocked down his own temple!

As the volume of literature in translation has increased, along with a sizable production of critical studies, the impact of Lacan's work on American psychoanalysis has continued to grow. It is still a modest influence, compared with the far more impressive notice given to Kohut, for example, who sometimes seems to govern the thought of the younger generation of analysts, and around whom fruitful controversies have developed. Partly this is due to the language; Kohut's books and papers appeared originally in a language that, although difficult, is still English, while Lacan comes to us as an exotic—some great, uncouth bear speak-

1. After writing the foregoing, I found the admirable article by Victor N. Smirnoff, "De Vienne à Paris" (1979), in which the author presents details of the history of psychoanalysis in France. While he shows that in the cases of René Laforgue and Edouard Pichon a French psychoanalysis had put in an appearance, with a singularly nationalistic inclination, the overriding influences were from the classical centers until the storm over Lacan broke. Smirnoff's account greatly enriches the scene, but it doesn't alter the perspective.

ing a combination of Mallarméan verse and French intellec-
tualese that turns into an English never before heard on land or
sea. Lacan also traveled under the cloud of his famous "excommunication," which by itself might actually rally support, save for
the fact that it appears to have been justified by his calamitous
technical procedures.

There is, however, something else to consider, a practical consideration: What difference might Lacan's theories make to *our*
clinical work? Lacan himself, it seems, could afford to brush aside
the question as impertinent, since he believed he had higher
aspirations (Turkel, 1978, p. 136), but for the clinician there are
no higher aspirations. Satisfying it may be indeed to have a newer
and keener insight into the minds of our patients, and especially
to be freed of the pseudobiological dependencies of the traditional libido theory or the occult tautologies that constitute much
of ego psychology; but how will this improve our work? We do not
ask for statistical evidence here but only for rational assurance
that we can do better work. I hope I may offer such assurance. My
purpose here is to look at Lacan as a contributor to the practice of
psychoanalysis as we know it.

Let me begin my discussion by quoting from a review of a book
about James Joyce. The reviewer mentions the influence of psychoanalytic and linguistic theory which, he summarizes,

> maintains that classic realistic fictions and conventional liter-
> ary criticism depend for their existence upon the notion of a
> unified conscious subject with confident and unquestioning
> access to the world of objects. Language is held to be a trans-
> parent means of reference to this world, especially in the case
> of the narratorial "meta-language" of the realist, that which
> judges other discourse and denies its own practices of con-
> structing meaning. But language can also be a threat to this
> easy correspondence. A heightened conception of its modes
> of operation and of the arbitrariness of its signs can lead us to
> fundamental questions about the production of meaning
> and our constitution as thinking subjects. [Brown, 1979]

These sentences, directed to be sure to literary criticism and
not to clinical or even theoretical psychoanalysis, could not have

been written except for the work of Jacques Lacan, among others. I must leave to the literary critics the now burning question whether this influence of psychoanalytic and linguistic theory is a stimulus to their discipline or a menace to its autonomy, or worse still to its intelligibility. The brief summary might rather serve here as an introduction to some of the deeper concerns of Lacanian analysis and how they might affect our work as psychoanalysts. Yet one cannot drop the matter of literary criticism without a further word: note how different this kind of psychoanalytic investigation of the text is from the older kind initiated by Freud (one might take "Delusion and Dream in Jensen's 'Gradiva'" as a starting point) and continued with increasing elaboration by all later practitioners of what he called "applied psychoanalysis." For them psychoanalytic criticism consisted in great measure of isolating from the literary text allusions to unconscious conflicts and relating these conflicts either to the fictional characters or to the author, or both. More sophisticated application of ego-psychological methods merely moved the locus of analysis closer to consciousness.

The newer psychoanalytic criticism has other intentions: it questions the assumptions on which the text is written—namely, that it means what it says and that the author knew what he or she meant. It proposes that the word and writing govern the writer and the reader. Heidegger's aphorism "Die Sprache spricht" comes into its own. Language, which we are accustomed to look on as an instrument for the communication of meaning, turns out to be its determinant. At the same time, all standards of objectivity are called into question. The speaker—or writer—is *spoken through;* he does not put his thought into words, but has his words thrust upon him. Correspondingly the reader—and here we might add, the listening analyst—is also not a "unified conscious subject" dealing with an external object. The situation seems anarchic, possibly chaotic, and silently paradoxical, because notwithstanding all this, the speaker or writer always is saying something and addressing it to somebody else.

It will be immediately apparent that what is at stake is our concept of the ego. There can be no quarrel with the position that the unconscious extends its dominion into all of conscious life.

Freud, not Lacan, subverted the Cartesian doctrine of the *cogito;*
if my being were inferrable from my conscious reflection alone,
who would be the agent intending my dream? Freud replied to a
similar question when he wrote that the dreamer is responsible
for his dream—who else could be? But in this affirmation he also
implies that the sleeping subject is either the agent of the primary
process or, as Lacan seems to prefer, its victim. Do we not hear
echoes (or perhaps see mirror images) of Groddeck's "It" to
which all conscious subjectivity submits its authority?

Prior to Lacan, Freudian theory had assumed a linear, although discontinuous, relationship between the unconscious subject and the conscious analysand—or between the analyst as unconscious subject and as conscious interpreter. Accordingly, the
conscious analysand and the analyst are, or can become, capable
of an objective recognition of the difference between the unconscious fantasy and the real world as defined by consensual consciousness. The distinctions between subject as initiator of the
dream (or other unconscious processes), subject as actor of the
dream, subject as speaker, subject as consciousness of self, subject
as agent of defensive distortion, subject as mediator between inner and outer world, and subject as discriminator between fantasy and reality—all these distinctions (I doubt that I have exhausted the possibilities) are present only in a blurred fashion.
They are blurred functionally, too, but the inadequacy of conceptual distinction has been misleading.

Lacan does not make the distinction exactly in this way, but
some such intention is implicit in his formulations. He wants
analysts to do away with the ego psychology which maintains this
inadequate conceptualization largely by conceiving of the ego as a
unitary structure equipped with "functions." He has an excep-
tionally lucid passage on this in his essay "The Freudian Thing."
He begins with a few jibes at the "burgraves" or feudal lords,
analysts who since around 1920 (and the publication of *The Ego
and the Id*) have allegedly stultified our work by their exaggerated
practice of the analysis of the resistance. (It is also characteristic of
Lacan that he exempts Freud from these jibes.) But "it is precisely
toward a reinforcement of the objectifying position in the subject

that the analysis of resistance was orientated"—that is, the more
we call attention to the resistance, the more we force the patient to
think about himself as an object, a thing among other things,
some part of which is to be removed. He continues,

> You cannot at the same time proceed yourself to this objec-
> tification of the subject and speak to him as you should. . . .
> That is, one's being cannot conform to two actions that lead
> in opposite directions. For, in psychology, objectification is
> subjected in its very principle to a law of *méconnaisance*
> [mis(re)cognition] that governs the subject not only as ob-
> served, but also as the observer. That is to say, it is not about
> him that you have to speak to him, for he can do this himself,
> and therefore, it is not even to you that he speaks. If it is to
> him that you have to speak, it is literally of something else,
> that is, of something other than that which is in question
> when he speaks of himself, and which is the thing that speaks
> to you, a thing which, whatever he says, would remain for-
> ever inaccessible to him, if in being speech [*parole*] addressed
> to you it could not elicit its response in you and if, from
> having heard its message in this inverted form, you could
> not, by returning it to him, give him the double satisfaction of
> having recognized it and of making him recognize its truth.
> [1977, p. 130]

In the same paper, Lacan makes the point more pithily:

> The prime condition . . . is that [the analyst] should be thor-
> oughly imbued with the radical difference between the
> Other to which his speech must be addressed, and the second
> other who is the individual that he sees before him, and from
> whom and by means of whom the first speaks to him in the
> discourse that he holds before him. For in this way, he will be
> able to be he to whom this discourse is addressed. [p. 140]

Not altogether easy statements, especially for one unfamiliar with
Lacan's mode of expression, the tortuosity of which does not
always bespeak profundity.

To explicate: as Lacan sees it, the "ego" means defensive distor-

tion. This distortion begins with the earliest placing of the subject
as a mirror image. The child's self-awareness is not a given but
comes from outside, literally from the reflection of the mirror,
but more important from the "specular" recognition of its existence as a "you" by the attending parents. Its "me" and later its "I"
are not autonomous, not even autogenous, so to speak, but are
conferred imputations. It is a gift with strings attached; because it
is derived from another's bounty, it is subject to another's caprice
(whence also the aggressivity of narcissism; see Lacan, 1977, p.
19). To be sure, prior to the "me" there is already an experiencing
subject, making itself known through its demands, originally
nonverbally, and, it seems, not even organized with respect to its
constituent body parts. This true subject is unconscious of self,
and when it has acquired language, speaks itself. On the other
hand, language too is a source of misrecognition. It is a gift of the
outside world, and being arbitrary, not matched to the requirements of the subject. Language is procrustean; it is not made to fit
individuals but fits the subject to itself. The full privacy of the
subject's own desire can become known only by the analysis of his
or her language.

One can see from this, I hope, the awkward position—to put it
mildly—of the interpreting analyst. It becomes still more awkward once we continue with Lacan to examine other aspects of
the situation, even if we stick to our familiar notions about transference. Who is speaking to whom, about what? Language, our
prized mode of communication, is demoted to a source of systematic misrepresentation. In the passage from Lacan that I have just
quoted, the misrepresentation is that of objectifying, seeing
oneself from a position prior to all defenses as a reasonable person after all, a *belle âme*, in Hegel's phrase. When the analyst
appeals to the so-called autonomous ego—a term that Lacan persistently derides—he is compounding the misrepresentation.
What passes for an autonomous ego is as much a defensive ma-
neuver as, for example, identification with the social role one is
supposed to execute. *Only the unselfconscious speaking of the patient
tells the truth.* Getting him to listen to reason is to reverse the
analytic process. This is the "radical difference" between the

"Other" (the unconscious subject of the patient's discourse) and the "other" (the patient as he presents himself to the analyst). Perhaps the important word is "radical": the disjunction between the conscious speaker and the unconscious subject is not something to be overcome by the famous "therapeutic alliance," for example. We do not by our interpretations of the ego defenses enlist on our supposedly rational side the supposedly rational aspect of the patient's ego. Yet all the while, it is the speaker, and only the speaker, who delivers the unconscious messages that it is the business of the analyst to decipher.

Taken in this extreme form (and it is only relatively extreme, since I am incapable of Lacan's gloriously hyperbolic expression), one might think that psychoanalysis has really become the "impossible profession" that Freud half-humorously declared it to be, but for a different reason from Freud's. It seems for Lacan that the establishment of any kind of rational discourse in the analysis runs counter to the exposure of the unconscious truth, and if there is no rational discourse, what then? There are at least three possible answers. First, the general experience of analysts over the decades, whatever our shortcomings, has not been entirely unsuccessful, and so we must have been doing something right. Second, if Lacan's argument is utterly persuasive we might have to try his method. Or third, the most to my liking, we can learn from Lacan's criticism and even accept much of his theoretical revision with possible improvement to our own method.

I would like to examine another side of Lacan's thought before proceeding further in an attempt to make our own what we can accept from him. This is the question of signification in connection with a fairly simple distinction between *word* and *theme*. If we conceive of the work of psychoanalysis as principally one of interpretation, we find that it proceeds along two paths. One, the thematic, consists of the assembling of ideas asserted by the analysand into structures unconsciously intended and presumed to bear latent meaning. Such meaning is presumed to exist not only in a single string of ideas but perhaps also in the ideas of a whole hour and sometimes even in a series of hours continuing for a long period. We might for example discern a predominantly positive oedipal theme which has been long hidden by its opposite. Another way to describe this part of the analytic work is to consider it the recognition of a series of unconscious fantasies that are fundamentally related. This relationship may be metaphoric, or paradigmatic, in the quality of partially substitutive overlap, or metonymic in the sense that the ideas are so closely associated that they derive meaning by their contiguity with one another. The important point is that when we infer thematic unities, we do so by disregarding the differences in their constituent appearances. We are defining a species of fantasy or theme by abstracting from the individual occurrences. At least in a phenomenological sense, this is a reduction, and perhaps also in a less attractive sense, if we introduce the notion that the theme is "nothing but" something other than its constitutive elements.

Although the thematic is only one aspect of analysis, I do not see how analysts could ever do without it entirely; we frequently need to be directed by general guidelines for the interpretation of unconscious content, which does, by any system justifying the name of Freudian analysis, submit to such formal thematic categories as the oedipal, the anal, the masochistic, and so forth. Indeed, Lacan, although as far as I can tell he does not encourage the interpretation of such categories, has himself introduced new categories (to supplement Freud rather than to supersede him, I believe), such as the specular, the primary signified, the master-slave dialectic, and others—not the least being "the Other"!

The second path of the interpretive work is the word, the concrete utterance. At first Lacan may seem to depart little from ordinary Freudian attention to words. He appreciates and persistently returns to Freud's "psychopathology of everyday life," to those instances where apparent verbal failure reveals unconscious intentions. There are numerous instances in Freud's writings in which the peculiarity of a word, such as a punning effect, literally signalizes the unconscious. Recall, for example, the Rat Man's repeated odd pronunciation of the conjunction *aber* with the accent strongly on the second syllable, leading Freud to suspect correctly that it concealed the word *Abwehr* (defense), which Freud had used while talking to him shortly before.

For Lacan such paronomasias are limitless. Indifferent-sound-

ing words are keys, by clang association, assonance, or some
other topical allusion, to the Other, that is, to the unconscious
subject. Lacan uses them himself in enunciating his ideas and he
hears them in practically any utterance. One must decide for
oneself to what extent this is mere cleverness or caprice, and its
use seems to me to call for some kind of discipline, lest it support a
wilder analysis than we have yet seen. There is a seductive inge-
nuity in a term such as "le Nom du Père," in which he implies the
fundamental symbolic role of the father. This allusive noun
phrase is itself drawn from the liturgic formula "in the name of
the Father, the Son and the Holy Spirit," the ironic tinge not
depriving it of all its hieratic association. But "le Nom du Père" is
also "le non du père," the father's command "No!," which for
Lacan ushers the symbolic world of law into the mind of the child.
Not content with this modest extrapolation of meaning, Lacan
has also insisted that "les non-dupes errent"—that nothing could
be more deceptive than thinking one is undeceived! On at least
one occasion he coyly referred to his women disciples as "les
nonnes du père," whereby he proclaims through a *mot* that he is—
as far as they are concerned—God, father, and the law.

We must remember that in the French tradition "preciosity"
(of which this last is a fine example) is not necessarily a disdainful
word but suggests an ear for nuance (a French word, too), developed to excess perhaps but still finely attuned to the implications
of words. Lacan's deliberate wordplay can be looked upon as
intellectual trickery if one takes his bait and becomes annoyed
with him. The theoretical basis of such playing with words is
found in Lacan's dictum that "the unconscious is structured like a
language." In his playful punning this claim is concretized, embodied. The unconscious can speak truthfully, revealing the
identity of logically unrelated, cognitively distorted, affectively
confused experiences. To the unconscious, things are what they
sound like. Paronomasia is only one of the tropes that reveal the
unconscious, but the others also do so by the universal property
of words as signifiers; they are arbitrary, and they derive their
meaning from their position in the total lexicon of a natural
language.

A clinical consequence is the extraordinary emphasis in Lacanian analysis on the specific words of the patient as distinguished, according to the dichotomy I have suggested, from the thematic path. We are familiar with this technical device, and usually warn our students to use it only sparingly and with the utmost care. The reasons for caution are sufficiently obvious—such playfulness may have the effect of seducing the patient by wit, diverting him to admire the preening analyst, or infuriating him with an implied put-down. With the Lacanians, it is a focus of treatment along with parapraxias, proper names that have special potency, and other tropes.

I have introduced and dwelt at some length on this aspect of Lacan's doctrine of signification because I think that despite the excessive use to which he evidently puts it, we may begin to see how it acts in opposition to the traditional position of the interpreting analyst. Although Lacan does use the words "drive" and "defense," he would hardly subscribe to our usual instruction to the student to interpret the defense and to turn to the drive only afterward. I remember being told as a beginner that I must look on the *id* as a simmering pot needing no assistance to boil over; it was all too ready to go, once I directed my attention, and my patient's, to the ego defenses. That instruction might really not be very far in effect from Lacan's allowing the unconscious to speak, but it is based on a different theoretical position. For Lacan it is a fatal flaw of the ego psychologists to look on defense as resistance, as something to be "worked through." Rather, it too is to be permitted to speak. Lacan's theoretical constructions are closer to a phenomenological stand than our traditional ones. Traditionally, we think that behind the word there is something else that is not word; the speaking side of analysis is epiphenomenon. Therefore some kind of formulational interpretation is in order, as though we could get behind and beyond the content of speaking to hidden hierarchies of thought, close to the conceptualizations by the analyst of the meaning of utterances.

Skilled analysts, in contrast to many beginners, do not look with favor on such interpretations, which smell of the library or even of the clinic. For example, an interpretive remark such as "You find yourself always retreating from people when you become emotionally involved with them" is not in itself horrendous, and may be a perfectly true description of someone's behavior, but as an interpretation it is an objectification, substituting for the living word of the patient a piece of knowledge, not for the subject as self, but of the subject as an imputed type—in Lacan's word, an "imaginary self" or even a thing. Contrast with it the following: the patient makes one of those curiously ambiguous remarks that in ordinary conversation are either overlooked or attributed to minor grammatical error, such as "I missed not seeing you when you were away." The "not" is a parapraxia, if we understand the speaker to mean that he consciously missed the analyst during vacation; but it is also, perhaps, a "knot" of another sort, a complex figure of ambivalences or a personal tie that cannot be loosened. An analytic procedure informed by Lacanian theory would, hypothetically, focus on the interpolated word rather than try immediately to formulate the affective situation. How the interpretation would be given is a highly individual matter; the possibilities might include a joking reference to the Gordian knot, or a gentler confrontation with the negative. The purpose in either case would be to encourage the patient to separate, and to utter, the meanings that are frozen in the nodal utterance (and the word "node" might be part of the pun, too).

Meaning, then, is saying, not formulating. And what is said is one's desire. Nothing could be more wrong than to think of Lacan's system as intellectualistic because of the insistence on words, on the "letter." The aim of all the wordplay is not to demonstrate the unconscious—any more than the ego—as a remarkable object inside the subject. It is to provide pathways for the speaking of desire. I shall not dwell here on Lacan's erratic and confusing distinction between demand and desire, although I do take for granted the important distinction of both from biological need. Desire, in particular, can be known only through the "defiles"— that is, the articulations—of the signifier, in words as part of a language. To be told, however convincingly, that one does thus and so because one loved one's sister at a certain time in childhood, as clearly manifested by a specific memory, is not the same as to utter, to speak, maybe to shout, in affect-laden words, right

now, that long-withheld desire. Lacan does not disown reference
to the past as some neo-Freudians do. On the contrary, his aim is
"rememoration," *le temps retrouvé,* so that the earlier loss is relived,
becomes conscious, in the statement of the patient of the present
instance of desire.

For Lacan everything is present in the words, including, of
necessity, the nonverbal, because words are the only way we can
get to the nonverbal. At the same time, we find the paradoxical
element that Lacan delights in: the patient's words and the analyst's interpretations never quite get to the point. An interpretation for Lacan is a kind of Zen *koan.* It is the opposite of what
Greenson (1967) seems to have had in mind when he wrote that
he aimed to be "simple, clear, concrete, and direct. I use words
that cannot be misunderstood." Greenson's intention was based
upon a linguistic notion foreign to Lacan. To "use words that
cannot be misunderstood" (which, to be sure, is a pretty big claim
by anyone's reckoning) is to assume a unitary connection between
word and idea or concept, so that when I say to my patient that
this means that, I am able to do so authoritatively. Interpretation
is supposed to impart positive knowledge by defining the quasi-
permanent signification of a fantasy or a series of associations. I
qualify with "quasi-" because a later review of the same associations in a new context, however slightly changed, may call for a
new definition.

The Lacanian view is really quite different. As a follower of
Saussure's structuralism, Lacan accepts the division of the verbal
sign into signifier and signified, word and concept. But the relation of signifier to signified is not "simple, clear, concrete, and
direct"; not only is it arbitrary, arising out of the discriminatory
lexicon of a natural language, but its meaning is burdened with
history and tinged by association. No signifying word can be uttered that does not have overlapping signification with other
words. The signified slides under the signifier. For the purposes
of interpretive technique, this means that the word of the analyst
matches the word of the patient not as signified but as another
signifier. Interpretation does not nail down meaning, it rings
bells, or, as I like to put it, interpretation aims not at closure but at
disclosure.

A simple illustration from everyday practice might be in order. The patient dreams about the eye, and from certain elements in the context of the analysis one might assume that the organ of vision is at issue, and a scopophilic wish intended. But one might also give thought to the possibility that the shifter-pronoun "I" is in question in the form of a rebus, and interpret accordingly—not of course by talking about the identity or any other abstraction, but by asking "Whose eye?" or "Who's 'I'?" This technique, of course, is not original—analysts have always used it, sometimes very badly, and with that deadly cleverness of which I spoke earlier. The difference is, first, the Lacanians lean far more exclusively on this technique of interpretation, and second, it illustrates the underlying linguistic theory as Lacan has appropriated it.[2]

In another instance, the parallel shifter-pronoun "we" led as a signifier into a host of rhetorical and semantic devices, not so much revealing as presenting fantasies of umbilical union, urinary incontinence, even the Platonic myth of the origins of sexuality. It led to the fantasy of the mirroring of the self, a kind of asexual reproduction, in the idea of shared fashions in clothing. Antithetically it disclosed the struggle to get the father's attention in order to interrupt the symbiotic bond, and in another direction it exposed the unconscious and violent opposition in the transference to any such interruption.

Such interpretations are probably easier than most, because of the intrinsic ambiguity of the pronouns as signifiers, although in both instances assonance and punning were independent of the shifting of referents. Ordinary substantives and verbs may lead to similar exposures as they are made to run through the same

---

2. A contemporary poet, Alfred Corn, uses the same trope:

An eye for an eye: the future darkens, goes blind.
I I I I—sounds like hammers, building
A barricade of rage. [1978, p. 40]

Just as Molière's M. Jourdain was surprised to learn that he had always been speaking prose, so our patients might be usefully surprised that, unconsciously, at times they speak verse!

variety of registers of signification. What is indispensable is alertness to the words as they appear, which paradoxically calls for a certain resistance on the analyst's part to our normal disposition to look for the *signified* concept, the theme.

I must leave it to my readers to decide whether the Lacanian concepts—the sliding of the signified under the signifier, the imaginary, the name of the father as law—are helpful in understanding the patient and making the unconscious *usefully* conscious. I think so, and I also claim that it is advantageous not to interpret in a "simple, clear, concrete, and direct" manner. What it will mean ultimately for the patient to speak his desire through the chain of signifiers that become disclosed in this fashion is not knowable. As I interpret—and doubtless modify—Lacan, the purpose is to help the patient to be confronted with the conflict in its depths and its breadth; it is perhaps more Heideggerian than Lacanian to add that this growth of consciousness of "being-in-the-world," especially the world of personal history and interpersonal concerns, is therapeutic.

The example I have offered of the analytic work influenced by Lacanian thinking has limitations. I have described only one facet of Lacan's complex system, but my purpose has been to suggest that one need not be a Lacanian to find useful technical applications of the system. I would not break a lance in defense of my point of view against those who contend that the same outcome can be reached by other routes, which is exactly what one might expect if the theory of the signifier is right: given world enough and time, the patient will say his meaning, will utter his desire. Kleinian, ego-psychological, object-relations theories, and probably others as well, might here converge, because whatever the analyst thinks, the patient must speak to be understood. Lacan has insisted that earlier methods of interpretive work delay or prevent utterance, because they locate meaning where it cannot be found, in the distortions of the ego. I believe that this criticism is no less applicable to the other theories than it is to the ego-psychological. Kleinian interpretations are disposed to reify the imaginary; the "bad breast" is a representation that can be spoken only symbolically, and to treat it as an ultimate signified is to fix it in the Imaginary.

And yet (there remains a big "and yet"), from what I have heard of Lacanian technique and some of its results, I am led to the conclusion that if applied consistently according to the precepts of Lacan, it must be as disposed to unsatisfactory outcome as any other technique. Even aside from Lacan's own exaggerations, there is a limit beyond which I would not want to go in the effort at the "subversion of the ego." To be consistent one would never say a logical sentence to the patient or listen to one from him or her. One would throw back words—if one spoke at all—rather as if they were lighted matches tossed at a powder keg, hoping for an explosion of a multiple meaning and rather likely to get one; but is this not again a reinforcement of long-held positions on the ego? To be sure, the patient will be surprised, perhaps at his own untapped possibilities but certainly at the analyst's omniscience. In addition, on several occasions when I have listened to some former analysands of Lacan's school I was impressed by how glibly they asserted their confirmation of theory—much as our own less successful patients do. In short, the duty of the independent analyst remains what it has always been: to bend consistency of theory to the exigencies of practice and to remain open to change of point of view.

I shall not close on a negative note. There is another way in which Lacan has affected psychoanalysis. As long as the basic structure of psychoanalysis was unchallenged within our own ranks, we approached that completion of our science which Eissler (1969) and probably others have promised—or maybe threatened. If we had settled down permanently with the libido theory, metapsychology, ego psychology, and the structural hypothesis, it is quite unlikely that anything unsettling would be heard from our patients, because we would have determined what we would hear and what we would ignore. When the emphasis is put on *speaking*, the science cannot be completed, and every new generation of analysts stands before a new world.

REFERENCES

Brown, J. Review of C. McCabe, *James Joyce and the Revolution of the World.* *Times Literary Supplement* (London), 21 December 1979.

Corn, A. *A Call in the Midst of the Crowd.* New York: Penguin, 1978.

Eissler, K. "Irreverent Remarks about the Present and the Future of Psychoanalysis." *International Journal of Psycho-Analysis* 50 (1969): 461–79.

Greenson, R. *The Technique and Practice of Psychoanalysis,* vol. 1. New York: International Universities Press, 1967.

Lacan, J. *Écrits: A Selection.* Translated by A. Sheridan. New York: Norton, 1977.

Leavy, S. "The Significance of Jacques Lacan." In J. H. Smith, ed., *Psychoanalysis and Language,* vol. 3 of *Psychiatry and the Humanities.* New Haven: Yale University Press, 1978.

Smirnoff, V. N. "De Vienne à Paris." *Nouvelle Revue de Psychanalyse* no. 20 (1979).

Turkel, S. *Psychoanalytic Politics.* New York: Basic Books, 1978.

Victor, G. "Interpretations Couched in Mythical Imagery." *International Journal of Psychoanalytic Psychotherapy* 7 (1978):225–39.

2

Language, Psychosis, and the Subject in Lacan

JOHN P. MULLER

The laws that structure the unconscious are identical to what Jakobson (1956) calls the principles of combination and substitution; they underlie all symbolic human action, and they are evident in dreams in the form of displacement and condensation. Thus, Lacan unequivocally states that

> the unconscious is structured in the most radical way like a language, that a material operates in it according to certain laws, which are the same laws as those discovered in the study of actual languages, languages that are or were actually spoken. [1977, p. 234]

One way to examine the import of this perspective is to consider, in a clinical example, the phenomenon of psychosis, for psychosis has always posed a critical challenge to any view of human existence. In 1946 Lacan stated: "Not only can man's being not be understood without madness, it would not be man's being if it did not bear madness within itself as the limit of his freedom" (1977, p. 215). This dictum may be understood as follows: it is our exposure to (and therefore possible foreclosure of) the symbolic order that defines both our being and our potential for madness. Now the symbolic order, for Lacan, has its own signifier: he calls it "the Name-of-the-Father," *le Nom-du-Père*, the signifier "which in the Other, as locus of the signifier, is the signifier of the Other as locus of the law" (1977, p. 221). The Name-of-the-Father, then, is the signifier of the pervasive law structuring human existence (in

French *nom* and *non* are homophonic) and the absence of this signifier "in the Other"—in the unconscious, that is—constitutes the structural defect in psychosis.

Its absence is a result not of repression, *Verdrängung*, but of foreclosure, which Freud himself distinguishes from *Verdrängung* by calling it *Verwerfung* (for detailed textual references in Freud, see Laplanche and Pontalis, [1967] pp. 166–69 and 390–94). What is repressed can be recovered and this is because a fundamental affirmation, a *Bejahung*, a registration of the repressed content in an unconscious symbolic text, has already occurred. In his Schreber essay (1977, p. 201) Lacan calls attention, in this context, to the semiotic implications of Freud's Letter 52 to Fliess (1896), in which he writes:

> As you know, I am working on the assumption that our psychical mechanism has come into being by a process of stratification: the material present in the form of memory-traces being subjected from time to time to a *re-arrangement* in accordance with fresh circumstances—to a *re-transcription* [*Umschrift*]. Thus what is essentially new about my theory is the thesis that memory is present not once but several times over, that it is laid down in various species of indications [*Zeichen* ("signs") says it much better]. [1950, p. 233]

Freud goes on to describe these levels of registration [*Niederschriften*], one of which he calls "*Wahrnehmungszeichen*," poorly translated as "indication of perception," since as "the first registration of the perceptions" it clearly has to do with perception being registered, unconsciously, writes Freud, under the rubric of "signs." The semiotic import for Freud is clear when he goes on to write of the "failure of translation [*die Versagung der Ubersetzung*]—this is what is known clinically as 'repression'" (1950, pp. 233–35; 1950b, pp. 185–87). Lacan makes explicit the linguistic nature of the unconscious registration of perceptions when he tells us, "We can immediately give to these *Wahrnehmungszeichen* their true name of signifiers" (1964, p. 46). Now in foreclosure no such *Bejahung* or affirmation has been made, no unconscious registration of the experience has occurred. This nonregistration Lacan contrasts to Heidegger's notion of *Seinlassen*, letting-something-be as disclosed being (1966, pp. 387–88). Foreclosure, then, is a refusal of such letting-be and a consequent cutting-short from manifestation in the symbolic order.

What experience is cut short here? For Lacan (as for Freud) it appears to be the experience of castration, of the mother's apparent castration as well as one's own. In psychotic development castration is foreclosed: the child remains in a dual, symbiotic union with the mother in which the child identifies with being the all-fulfilling object of the mother's desire. For Lacan, the signifier of the mother's desire is the phallus. Thus, in attempting to *be* the imaginary phallus or completion of the mother the child rejects the limits implied by castration. These limits are the constraints invoked by the Law of the Father, the symbolic father who intervenes in this dual relation, establishes primal repression by structuring desire according to the laws of language, and makes it possible for the child to have a place in a signifying network of kinship relations, sex roles, sanctions, and discourse. When the mother fails to affirm the Law of the Father, makes no room for the intervening role of the symbolic father, or when the real father himself has a hypocritical relation to the Law, the Name-of-the-Father as signifier is foreclosed, and therefore the symbolic castration involved in giving up the position of the phallus and becoming subject to the Law is also foreclosed (for an excellent example of the mother's role in this, see De Waelhens [1972], pp. 62–66). Lacan describes this as the failure of the paternal metaphor (1977, p. 215), the failure of the Name-of-the-Father to substitute for the Desire-of-the-Mother and inaugurate the structure of primal repression in which the phallus goes below the bar and functions as the unconscious signifier of desire.

The actual psychotic episode that may occur in later life is triggered in a transferencelike encounter with what Lacan terms "A-Father," a father figure in a special relationship to the subject (for Schreber, of course, this figure was his physician, Flechsig). The encounter with A-Father invokes the fundamental signifier of the father, but since it has been foreclosed, there is only a hole, a gap, in the symbolic order where this signifier should be. The experience of this hole in the signifying realm sets off a desperate attempt to fill it through the imaginary reshaping of signifiers and a fundamental alteration of previous signifier-signified relationships, leading to narcissistic delusions and a loss of consensually validated speech. In attempting to *be* the phallus, the psychotic typically struggles with having or not having the phallus: thus, Schreber's delusion centered on the imaginary-real castration implied in his becoming a woman, his not having the phallus in order to *be* God's phallus.

In another clinical example, a male patient—call him Patrick— was in his twenties when he came for long-term treatment after previous hospitalizations occasioned by a schizophrenic break in high school. His psychosis was marked by delusions, clanging speech, suicidal panic, intermittent homicidal thoughts, and a belief that people were calling him homosexual. Since early puberty he had been essentially isolated, keeping to his room and TV during nonschool hours, avoiding contact with his father. Patrick never dated but made brief attempts at college, only to return home, where he experienced frequent anxiety attacks and ideas of reference regarding TV, radio, and phonograph messages. He shared these anxious moments with his mother during daily afternoon talks on the porch.

In the early months of long-term treatment Patrick gradually weaned himself from an incoming daily dose of almost two grams of Thorazine. He spoke of being both fascinated and troubled by words, which he would break apart and put together to form new ones. At times he would stumble over conjunctions; for example, when he used "but" his mind would think of "smoke a butt," "smoked butt," and of making fun of someone, like the homosexual joking in high school. When anxious he would have fantasies of cutting off his penis and recalled how the boys used to call him "she." One night he asked if he could have his Thorazine and was told "You surely may." Thinking the nurse had called him a "Surely may," he became anxious. "A girl's name?" the therapist asked. "No, I didn't think of it that way," he said; "just as an object." He recalled that when riding in the car with his father, he would play with a dictionary, looking up the meaning of one word, then looking up the meaning of a word used in defining the first, and so on. "Words unconsciously change their meaning for me," he said. He spent weeks obsessed with ideas about mental cannibalism, in which his words were taken in by others, and he began to say a fixed prayer, provided by his mother, to stop the anxiety attacks. He also began to take notes on his thoughts during anxiety states and bring them into therapy to read: "Haven't *been* saying the prayer." "*Bean* as in head." "*Head* as in penis." "Made me" and "Madame."

Six months into treatment Patrick was completely off medication, had adjusted well to hospital routines, had taken up painting, and was able to describe some of the events that led to his first psychotic episode. At that time in a high school course on myth and philosophy he was impressed by the instructor's breadth of culture and oratorical style (unlike, he said, his father's businesslike speech). The instructor's son was also taking the course and Patrick was impressed by the free-and-easy relations he observed between father and son. At the start of the course the instructor was emphasizing the subjective nature of perception and pointed to Patrick, saying "*You* are the center of the universe." At the end of the course, nine weeks before the psychotic break, the instructor wrapped things up by asking, "Now, *who* did I say was the center of the universe?"

After ten months of open-hospital treatment the patient's sexual interest in one of his therapist's female patients was rebuffed. At about the same time he met the therapist's wife and toddler son at a patient-staff picnic. There then rapidly developed a month-long resurgence of psychotic symptoms. Patrick thought his speech was Shakespearean, that he was Superman, St. Patrick, and could influence others and the weather through electromagnetic forces. His mood shifted from the euphoria that came with being able to understand and feel everything—which is typical of psychotic states—to an empty despair marked by angry outbursts over the insincere speech of staff and patients.

During his sessions he was often incoherent, would become angry when the therapist failed to comprehend his words, and

was fixated on his own hand gestures and on any slight movements of the therapist, which he would mimic. Once while his
parents were away he went home and drove his father's car back,
stopping for a day in a nearby city. As he walked around he felt
that the entire city was joyously celebrating his arrival—the arrival of God—and that everyone was aware of his feelings. Back at
the hospital he was convinced that he had the power to change the
car radio's dial setting with his thoughts and demanded that the
therapist sit in the car to observe this phenomenon. Refusing to
give up the car keys, he became more and more a management
problem; he was asked to go back on medication but rejected it
three days later. After he threatened to assault a staff member,
the staff thought he might have to be transferred to a closed
hospital.

At that point two visiting graduates of Lacan's school who re-
viewed the case suggested that the therapist make two interventions: that Patrick be firmly told that to mingle his body with the
other patient's was absolutely forbidden, and that he should be
asked to bring some of his paintings into a therapy session. At the
appropriate moments the prohibition and the invitation were
given by the therapist. Patrick initially responded angrily to the
prohibition, but then said he realized it was necessary "because
we're so alike that if we had sex one of us would be snuffed out."
As for the paintings, he initially invited the therapist to come see
them in his room. When the therapist refused and repeated the
invitation that Patrick bring some into a session, he came in with
twenty or so, laid them out on the floor, described their colors,
and recollected his feelings while painting them; he left some in
the office and as he ended the session said, "Say, maybe tomor-
row we can stop the double-talk." Turmoil continued, but three
weeks after the interventions, without the aid of medication, the
overt psychosis rapidly diminished, whereupon Patrick became
quite depressed. Over the second year of treatment he gradually
began to socialize more, was not overtly psychotic, continued
painting, and remained off medication.

While we cannot be certain about causal efficacy in this kind of
work, we can attempt to situate what happened in a Lacanian

framework, where the psychotic state is viewed as one of immediacy in which the patient is "glued" to the bodily presentation of
the therapist and where words no longer serve to mediate relationships but function rather as objects. In this boundless, grandiose state interpretations are at best meaningless and at worst
provocative. Caught in this immediacy, the patient experiences at
once a kind of ecstasy and horror, and his eventual options are to
kill the other (primarily the parasitic mother of the symbiosis) or
to kill himself and thereby be liberated from this monstrosity. In
this context how can we understand the function of the interventions?

The prohibition against mingling bodies attempted to affirm
the limits of the patient's body in the face of threatened bodily
fragmentation and boundlessness; it also introduced a lack, a *no*,
a limit to the grandiosity. The invitation, on the other hand,
attempted to open a transitional space between patient and therapist within the framework of the therapy—a kind of third dimension that is not part of the unmediated real, nor captivating like
an image, but not yet actually symbolic, not part of the symbolic
order of interpretation or discourse from which the patient had
lost his fragile moorings. The paintings, it was hoped, would
serve as presignifying transitional objects that would cut the
bonds of immediacy between patient and therapist and allow for
the emergence of new modes of signifying. Indeed, three months
after the interventions, as Patrick described one of the paintings
he had shown, he said it represented his feelings of being defec-
tive and expressed "my pain, like castration."

Another way to explore the role of the interventions (and the
reader may consider yet other frameworks) is provided by the
linguistic paradigm discussed earlier: the prohibition, as limit,
reestablishes contiguity and thus the conditions of possibility for
metonymy as a displacement of desire. The invitation to bring in
the paintings, in turn, opens an arena for substitution (the therapist's office for the patient's room, the paintings for words) and
thus reestablishes the conditions for spoken metaphor as intrinsically comporting a repressed dimension.

Much good and bad has been written about the characteristics of psychotic speech. A recent Danish study of letters and transcribed interviews of psychotic patients, using a Lacanian framework, found "disorders characterized by metonymical slidings of the signifier" and a replacement of the second person addressed with a grandiose, fantasized Other. The structured anchoring of "I" and "you" within the symbolic order gives way to a blurring of body boundaries, with the result that "metonymic slidings dominate the text: words and even sentences seem to be substituted according to the law of the signifier rather than to the logic of the signified" (Rosenbaum and Sonne, 1979, p. 4), as typified in the frequently observed clang associations of the psychotic. Thus, Lacan sees this as a "discourse in which the subject, one might say, is spoken rather than speaking" (1977, p. 69).

In a certain sense the speaking subject is "overthrown," for the psychotic no longer lives in a world mediated by language. He lives "in the real," in immediacy. The real has no gaps or lacks, and this absence of lack (if that can be conceived) is the inverse of what goes on in signification. Lacan tells us the word is "a presence made of absence" (1977, p. 65). Lack is intrinsic to the signifier as signifier. When we speak or read a word, we do not stop at the mere sound or drops of ink (unless we are psychotic). We see through the word *to* another that is absent. This absent other is, first of all, all the other words as the background against which the word has salience. Second, we see through the word as signifier to its retrospective and prospective impact on the other words in the sentence. Third, we are given in the word the symbolic presence of what is signified. The word *refers*, it is never taken simply in itself substantively. It has no substance in itself, except as a kind of medium that always comports an *other*, many others; it always slips equivocally and referentially along a polyphonic multiregister that establishes multileveled resonances. The real, on the contrary, is a kind of static whole as well as a kind of black hole void of internal relations. To "live in the real" means then to experience not just "loss of self" but an unbearable plenitude; the term "jouissance" catches the ecstatic quality of it but not the horror. An often used example of this horror is the classical Greek view of the unburied corpse stuck in the real—the rotting, fragmenting corpse that haunts the survivor until appropriate funeral rites can be carried out so that the grave of the deceased can receive a marker, a signifier, and the reality of death can then be inscribed in the symbolic order and thereby be repressed and forgotten. Without the signifier there is no repression.

In the psychotic state, there is no distance or perspective on experience, there is no "cut," no repression, and therefore no true signifier-signified relationship. The symptom no longer signifies but is lived, a metaphor lived as real. Words do not mediate, do not refer to what is absent, but function in the real as objects (akin to Freud's analysis of schizophrenia as cathexis of the *Wortvorstellung* in place of the *Sachvorstellung* [1915, pp. 197–204]).

Lacan tells us, following Hegel, that the word is "the murder of the thing" (1977, p. 104). The word destroys the immediacy of objects, and gives us distance from them, by making them present in speech, by transforming what is physically at hand or physically absent into what is symbolically present. It is the symbolic presence effected by words that both makes possible the toleration of absence and provides us with substitute objects of desire. Freud expressed this in his example of the child's *Fort! Da!* game, in which play with the spool tied to a string in conjunction with the phonemes *o-o-o!* and *da!* marks his moment of separation from his mother, a moment in which, Lacan tells us, desire becomes human and the child is born into language. It is precisely here that Winnicott's notion of the transitional object has relevance, and a relevance acknowledged by Lacan himself when he introduces it in the context of the child's emerging from need into the realm of desire (1977, p. 312). For Winnicott, transitional phenomena belong to neither inner nor outer reality but to "the third part of the life of a human being" (1971, p. 2), an "intermediate state" (p. 3) in which the infant passes from omnipotent, magical control to manipulative-motor control (p. 9). In this realm the transitional object provides a "neutral area of experience which will not be challenged" (p. 12). In further defining "the transitional object," Winnicott writes:

> It is not the object, of course, that is transitional. The object represents the infant's transition from a state of being merged with the mother to a state of being in relation to the mother as something outside and separate. [pp. 14–15]

Lacan crucially adds, of course, that in the *Fort! Da!* game the mother is now able to be present in her absence through words, and he thus completes Winnicott's conception. For the transitional object is not yet a signifier—Lacan calls it "le représentant de la représentation" (1966), p. 814), only an emblem, perhaps akin to Freud's *Vorstellungsrepräsentanz,* which serves to fix drive to its representative and thereby establish primal repression and, through repression, the unconscious (see Laplanche and Pontalis, pp. 203–05).

Now this is just what is at stake in psychosis: transitional phenomena are aborted; they do not yield toleration of separation and the signification of absence. The "paternal metaphor" has not taken hold and therefore there is no stable structure of primal repression. Instead, the patient has learned, before the first psychotic break, to mask the structural gap, to conceal (with the family's connivance) the foreclosure of the fundamental signifier of the Father that ordinarily substitutes for the Desire-of-the-Mother and makes possible genuine participation in the symbolic order. The symbolic castration required by the Law of the Father, which intervenes in the dual relation between infant-as-phallus and mother's desire, establishes the price one pays for becoming a subject—subject to the law of language which henceforth structures human desire through metaphor and metonymy. The earlier Heideggerian note can now have its complete relevance. The process of *Seinlassen,* letting-something-be, is fully achieved only in language, "the house of Being" (Heidegger, 1947, p. 193) whereby things come to presence through words (for further elaboration, see Richardson [1963], pp. 216, 496–97). It is, then, through the generation of a signifier in transitional space that the psychotic patient can effectively register his experience, transform its immediacy by giving it a presence in words, and become subject therefore to the structure of language.

This structure radically determines our lives as human subjects, as subject to its Law: it subjects us to primordial loss, the loss of fantasized totalization in symbolic castration, the loss incurred in separation from the immediacy of maternal symbiosis, the loss of that part of ourselves and our desire that henceforth finds expression only in the bits and pieces of metaphoric substitution and an unending metonymic displacement. To be finitely human means to live as decentered subjects, split and barred from unconscious desire, forced to channel our wants through the narrow defiles of the signifier, which offers a limited satisfaction by affording us symbolic presences. The alternative is either death or psychosis, where there is neither presence nor absence and no speaking subject.

REFERENCES

De Waelhens, A. *Schizophrenia: A Philosophical Reflection on Lacan's Structuralist Interpretation* (1972). Translated by W. Ver Eecke. Pittsburgh: Duquesne University Press, 1978.

Freud, S. *Standard Edition of the Complete Psychological Works*. London: Hogarth, 1955–74.
"Psycho-analytic Notes on an Autobiographical Account of a Case of Paranoia (Dementia Paranoides)" (1911), vol. 12.
"The Unconscious" (1915), vol. 14.
"Extracts from the Fliess Papers" (1950 [1892–99]), vol. 1.
————. *Gesammelte Werke*. London: Imago, 1942–43. "Psychoanalytische Bemerkungen Über Einen Autobiographisch Beschriebenen Fall von Paranoia (Dementia Paranoides)" (1911b), vol. 8.
————. *Aus den Anfängen der Psychoanalyse: Briefe an Wilhelm Fliess, Abhandlungen und Notizen aus den Jahren 1887–1902*. Edited by M. Bonaparte, A. Freud, and E. Kris. London: Imago, 1950b.

Heidegger, M. "Letter on Humanism" (1947). Translated by F. Capuzzi and J. G. Gray. In *Basic Writings*. Edited by D. F. Krell. New York: Harper & Row, 1977.

Jakobson, R. "Two Aspects of Language and Two Types of Aphasic Disturbances." In R. Jakobson and M. Halle, *Fundamentals of Language*. The Hague: Mouton, 1956.

Lacan, J. *The Four Fundamental Concepts of Psycho-Analysis* (1964). Edited by J.-A. Miller. Translated by A. Sheridan. New York: Norton, 1978.
————. *Écrits*. Paris: Seuil, 1966.

————. *Écrits: A Selection.* Translated by A. Sheridan. New York: Norton, 1977.

Laplanche, J., and Pontalis, J.-B. *The Language of Psychoanalysis* (1967). Translated by D. Nicholson-Smith. New York: Norton, 1973.

Richardson, W. J. *Heidegger: Through Phenomenology to Thought* (1963). Preface by M. Heidegger. The Hague: Martinus Nijhoff, 1967.

Rosenbaum, B., and Sonne, H. *Summary of* Det er et bånd der taler *[It is a tape that speaks]: Analysis of Language and Body in Psychosis.* Copenhagen: Gyldendals Sprogbibliotek, 1979.

Winnicott, D. W. *Playing and Reality.* New York: Basic Books, 1971.

3

Within the Microcosm of "The Talking Cure"

Julia Kristeva

It would be strange for a psychoanalyst, asked to present her own reading of Jacques Lacan's texts and practice, to consider herself either a propagator or a critic of his work. For the propagation of psychoanalysis—a conflictive, imaginative activity based on the unknown and on a specific manifestation of the individual unconscious—has shown us, ever since Freud, that interpretation necessarily represents appropriation, and thus, an act of desire and murder.

In the following pages, I will first try to present one possible reading—my own—of Lacan's contributions to the interrelations between language and the unconscious. This problematic, central to his work, has undoubtedly been influenced not only by his association with literary avant-garde movements of the thirties (Surrealism and its successors), but more significantly, by his profound interest in psychosis.[1] In the second half of my presentation, I will suggest, on the basis of this critical reading of Lacan, an

Translated by Thomas Gora and Margaret Waller.

Part of this essay has been published in French as "Il n'y a pas de maître a langage," in *Regards sur la psychanalyse en France*, a special issue of *Nouvelle Revue de la psychanalyse* (Autumn 1979); the second part was the topic of a seminar I delivered at the Centre Hospitalier Sainte Anne in the spring of 1981.

1. See Lacan's doctoral thesis, *De la psychose paranoïaque dans ses rapports avec la personnalité* (1932) (Paris: Seuil, 1975), followed by his *Premiers écrits sur la paranoïa*, also written in the thirties.

analytical attentiveness both to the discourse of borderline patients and to the types of interpretation it elicits from the analyst.[2]

The Heterogeneous

Critiques of Lacanian theory have included a number of attempts to give status to affect and to the heterogeneity it introduces into the discursive order. I have suggested elsewhere that
the language object be considered, on a semiological level, as a
"process of signifiance" in which the heterogeneity of two separate
modes should be distinguished: the *semiotic,* emanating from instinctual drives and primary processes; and the *symbolic,* assimila-
ble to secondary processes, predicative synthesis and judgment;
and I have posited the logical and chronological priority of the
symbolic in any organization of the semiotic (into a structure but
also a "chora," a receptable).[3]

Lacan's notion of *lalangue,* "the-so-called-mother-tongue,"
which dates from his seminar of 1972–73, introduced a fundamental refinement into the relation between the unconscious and
language previously elaborated. As something completely different from communication or dialogue, as the domain of equivoca-
tion and *Witz, lalangue* was to represent the real from which linguistics takes its object: "Language is what we try to know about
the functioning of *lalangue.*"[4] This formulation must be dis-

2. See D. W. Winnicott, "Ego Distortion in Terms of True and False Self"
(1960), in *The Maturational Processes and the Facilitating Environment: Studies in the
Theory of Emotional Development* (New York: International Universities Press,
1965).

3. See J. Kristeva, *La Révolution du langage poétique* (Paris: Seuil, 1974), "L'Hét-
érogène." To support this notion of a *semiotic chora,* we could view *instinctual drive*
less as a "figure" (a term to be reserved for a phenomenology of consciousness,
which Husserl demonstrates is indistinctly linked to spatiality) than as "uncou-
plings, fragmentations, dislocations, decompositions, and ruptures, but also
closures." This leads us to think of the unconscious as "coming about and immo-
bilizing itself within a logic of the psychic body" (J.-B. Pontalis, *Entre le rêve et la
douleur;* Paris: Gallimard, 1977, p. 250), which for us is always a translinguistic
phenomenon.

4. J. Lacan, *Encore* (Paris: Seuil, 1975), p. 126.

tinguished from his previous one ("The unconscious is structured like a language"). For if "language . . . is the fact of *lalangue*" or even "laborious intellectual work on *lalangue*," then the
unconscious cannot be reduced to it because, although language
is of course "knowledge," it is "a *savoir-faire* with *lalangue*. And
what we know how to do with *lalangue* [*ce qu'on sait faire avec
lalangue*] is far more than what we can account for under the
heading of language." "If we can say that the unconscious is
structured like a language, it is because the effects of *lalangue*,
which are already there as knowledge, go far beyond what any
speaking being can utter."[5] This idea seems to threaten the impe-
rialism of utterance and enunciation to such a degree that *lalangue* is definitely animated by affects that involve the presence
of nonknowledge: "These affects result from the presence of
lalangue, in so far as it articulates things about knowledge far
beyond what the speaking being can bear to know are uttered."[6]

Lalangue is undoubtedly coherent with the rest of Lacan's theory because, while the concept assigns to "language" (as an object
of linguistics and of such subordinate categories as "language,"
"speech," "discourse," "utterance," "act of enunciation," etc.) the
realm of *signification, lalangue* integrates the realm of *meaning
[sens]* into the field of psychoanalysis; and although the realm of
meaning is never totalizable and is continually perforated by non-
sense, it is nevertheless *homogeneous* with the realm of signification, even going so far as to assimilate what the dualism in Freudian thought regarded as strangely irreducible: instinctual drive,
affect. No matter how impossible the *real* might be, once it is made
homogeneous with *lalangue*, it finally becomes part of a topology
with the *imaginary* and the *symbolic*, a part of that trinary hold
from which nothing escapes, not even the "hole," since it too is
part of the structure.

The problem of the heterogeneous in meaning, of the unsym-
bolizable, the unsignifiable, which we confront in the analysand's

5. Ibid., p. 127.
6. Ibid. See the commentary on *lalangue* by J.-A. Miller in *Ornicar* 1 (1975):
16–34, and J.-Cl. Milner, *L'Amour de la langue* (Paris: Seuil, 1978).

discourse as an inhibition, a symptom, or an anxiety, characterizes the very condition of the speaking being, who is not only split
but split into an irreconcilable heterogeneity. And this problem
still remains unresolved. To keep it unresolved not only is the
condition of *jouissance* for the analyst, but also guarantees that the
cure will not become a safety net whereby the subject would believe himself master of *lalangue*, if not of language. Freud's pessi-
mism obviously comes to mind here, and Lacan's as well when he
resigns himself to designating by "sinthome" that which is irre-
ducible-to- signifiance, which the word *lalangue* might lead us to
believe can be transformed into thought, mathemes, or words.[7]

I would insist, however, that language's or *lalangue*'s "irre-
ducibility-to-a-signifier" is nonetheless translinguistic: it exists
and can be conceived only through the *position*, the thesis, of
language. For to imagine the autonomy of the "trace," the "picto-
gram," or the "cryptogram" with respect to language's own thetic
position, or to envisage some logical or chronological precedence
to its impact, would be to give a helping—that is, a theoretical—
hand to the maintenance of the notion of the maternal phallus;
we would also be encouraging narcissistic regression—a jubilation of specular echoes as the ultimate goal of the cure.

Furthermore, the position of the semiotic as heterogeneous
does not derive from a desire to integrate, within a language
often accused of being too "abstract," a supposed concreteness, a
raw corporeality, or an immanent energy. To posit, as such, concrete and intuitive purities is undoubtedly a fantasm that appeals
to medical rationality, which views language only for what it
transmits as a reality principle—that is, (de)negation. On the contrary, as Hegel already knew, and as any analyst with ears can

7. Lacan coined the word "sinthome" in reference to Joyce ("Joyce et le sinthome") and in the image of its old spelling ("symtome"). The neologism allows
him, in the Joycean context, to include within the notion of symptom an allusion to
sin and to St. Thomas as well. It is a hint at the presence of theology in Joyce but
also perhaps in analytic experience itself.

"Matheme" is a mathematical term. In his formalization of discourse on the
subject, Lacan turns to topology, among other things. Is it a symbolic or an imaginary tool? Lacanians debate the matter, but Lacan seemed rather to be having fun
with it.

hear, it is the very process of abstraction and logic which gives us access to the most essential, the most hidden concreteness.

Nevertheless, we still have the problem of differentiating, within the flow of discourse, *modes of articulation* and *types of logic*. Why? So as to hear in what is said where it suffers and where there is *jouissance*—not only through the different *figures* or *spaces* made by those signs which resemble linguistic signs, but also through *other elements* (Freud's "instinctual representatives" and "perceptual traces," etc.) which, although always already caught in the web of meaning and signification, are not caught in the same way as the two-sided units of the Saussurean sign and even less so in the manner of linguistico-logical categories. Thus the *semiotic chora* gives a different status to "signifying" marks: heterogeneous, mobile, dynamic; material traces and distinctive marks; the possibility of condensation and displacement as articulations; places of *jouissance* (when it undermines the signifier/signified distinction and predicative synthesis) and of defense (when it becomes blocked).[8] Thus this semiotic mode has no primacy, no point of origin. When I hear it in echolalias, intonations, irrecuperable

8. We should keep in mind the incredible complexity of Freud's notion of a "sign," which is exorbitant compared with the closure imposed on the sign by Saussure's stoicism. The Freudian "sign" is outlined in *On Aphasia: visual, tactile,* and *acoustic* images linked to object associations which refer, principally through an auditory connection, to the *word* itself, composed of an *acoustic* and *kinesthetic* image, of *reading* and *writing*. The fact that the *acoustic* image is privileged in this case does not diminish the heterogeneity of this "psychological blueprint of word-presentations," which today we still have difficulty assimilating, even with the rigor of linguistics and analytical attentiveness. And yet, the nature of this "imagery" will remain incomprehensible unless we perceive it as always already *indebted* (in a more or less "primary" or "secondary" way, as he would later say) to that representability specific to language, and therefore to the linguistic *sign* (signifier/signified). While this sign serves as the internal limit upon which Freud structures his notions of *presentation* and *cleavage* (what Lacan makes explicit in his "linghysteria"), it is by no means the most far-reaching of Freud's discoveries. Freud's conception of the unconscious derives from a notion of language as both heterogeneous and spatial, outlined first in *On Aphasia* when he sketches out as a "topology" both the physiological underpinnings of speech ("the territory of language," "a continuous cortical area," "centers" seen as *thresholds,* etc.) as well as language acquisition and communication (the after-word, the relation to the Other). See J. Nassif, *Freud, l'Inconscient* (Paris: Galilée, 1977).

ellipses, asyntactical and alogical constructions—in all of these divergences from codified discourse, but also in gestures, laughter and tears, moments of acting out—the semiotic chora appears within the signifying *process* as the trace of the *jouissance* that the subject gives himself with the other, with or through language itself, protecting himself from the lost territories, uncontrollable and overflowing, that elude the incisiveness of predicative synthesis and judgment and that he imagines to be his body—that is, always the body of that subject, the body of this subject speaking that discourse.

We should reread "Negation" once again. It reminds us that already in Freud, if (de)negation permits thought, and thus if desexualization or a desire for repression constitutes both judgment and the language that is its locus, (de)negation, thought, speech also constitute sex. (De)negation, like the speech act articulated in it, represents an undecidable tension, an *interval* between heterogeneous opposites, an "uncanny," which the analyst alone, and not the linguist, seeks to bring out. Here, in this undecidability, lies the analyst's desire and his ethics. That is why (de)negation (negation? speech?: Freud remains within the undecidable) is a progression toward the infinite coming into consciousness of the repressed. Last, and not insignificant, this negativity, which both brings into being (within discourse) the desire that discourse deflects and brings to consciousness what is repressed in speech, is nothing more than a stasis in instinctual drive, in the death instinct, under the effects of the paternal interdiction. Language is the terrain of death work: this is what should be heard when language represses (displaces, repulses, expels, and supplants); or when it brings desire into being through its very structure, which is that of (de)negation—the lapses or failures of language being merely the symptoms of (de)negation. Like the "no" from which it derives, language signals repression while at the same time releasing pleasure. The death instinct finds in language its master, but the analyst's task is to hear the slave behind the master, who, because of him, suffers and experiences pleasure: desire, death . . . .

Such an analysis of the position of thought and of language, which is coextensive with thought, reveals the perverse economy by which they are sustained. To the projective identification mechanism that Melanie Klein's followers see as presiding over the birth and functioning of the symbol, we could add the perverse implications for symbolization in language deriving from (de)negation. The analyst who takes this into account probably will not assume the pleasurable role of comforting or persecuting mother; instead he will hold on to the thread guiding him through this game of hide-and-seek or chess, which is the narrow path of transference and countertransference intermingled with sex and death. The analyst's attentiveness to language makes him open to works of art, since it is so-called aesthetic production that *knows how to deal with [sait faire avec]* the (de)negation inherent in language, without actually knowing it. Aesthetic production knows how to bring its perverse economy to *jouissance,* thereby deferring the castration and death that the analyst, by contrast, is continually trying to pinpoint.

Finally, to understand unconscious discourse it seems essential to maintain the thetic and organizing role of the object *language,* as contemporary linguistics defines it, so that from and through language there can emerge in the process of signifiance what remains irreducible to language—that is, its real. For therein lies, precisely, the specific object of the analyst's attentiveness. We must therefore remain attentive to recent developments in the *linguistics of enunciation,* which, without overturning that discipline's phenomenological foundations, deciphers meaning in light of intersubjective relations within the discursive act (for example, the logic of *presupposition,* its particularities in *interrogative discourse,* and so forth, which allow us better to discern a "preconscious logic" as distinct from the logic of unconscious effraction). Certain changes in the field of linguistics itself are related to this analytical interrogation of signifiance. Thus, when semantic and syntactic research questions the pertinence of grammatical categories, replacing them with the articulation of semantic traits whose value is not immanent but "merely" a function of their *position,* this may well be a decisive step in going beyond the Cartesian subject as the subject of a linguistic enunciation.

Moreover, since this linguistics of enunciation is attentive to enunciative phenomena such as *intonation,* which until now have only been considered secondary in the description of utterance, it is discovering that intonation is far more than the carrier of a summons or emotional expressivity; it is an archaic component (in language acquisition) of *syntax,* just as it is essential in removing the ambiguity of any utterance (constituting syntactic and semantic identity) which is caught in the act of communication. Intonation, a fundamental factor of language usually considered more closely linked to instinctual drive and the unconscious, is, according to recent research, largely integrated within syntactic structure. This poses problems for linguistics, forcing it either to posit between "primary" (semantic) and "secondary" (phonological) articulations a third or *prosodical* articulation (which integrates morphemes and sentences), or else to revamp completely the stages it envisages between "form" and "meaning."[9] That linguistics is broadening its field by taking as its object not only language but discourse as an act of enunciation does not, however, mean that linguistics is treating the unconscious phenomena of enunciation as well.[10]

This discipline's horizon is still phenomenology and its transcendental ego, whose *intention*—indeed, its *intuition*—never goes beyond the thesis of *meaning* and *form.* While it is true that we can enunciate nothing that does not stumble up against this transcendental horizon of meaning and form, analytical discourse or the discourse of the analysand since Freud has made us see that those are, precisely, only *stumbling blocks,* through which, against which, there operates an irreducible heterogeneity, ever elusive and divisive, but qualitatively other. Libido, desire, instinctual drive, affect: it goes by various names according to the conceptual framework of the theory that posits it and the level of its operations. But the name always designates something irreducible, a disquieting heterogeneousness, outside the transcendental en-

9. See the discussion on intonation in the *Bulletin de la Société linguistique de Paris,* no. 72 (1977).

10. On this question, some linguists believe that a large part of enunciative phenomena do not enter into semantic and syntactic construction, but instead remain unconscious. Ibid., p. 9.

closure within which we are otherwise constrained by phenomenology and its relative, linguistics.

Two Types of Interpretation in the Cure of a Borderline Patient: Construction and Condensation

In analytical practice we find discourses which at the outset of the cure seem to be borderline or neurotic but which, after a while and through an extreme attentiveness, prove to derive from a bizarre disarticulation of the language function.[11] Beneath the seemingly well-constructed grammatical aspects of these patients' discourse we find a futility, an emptying of all affect from meaning—indeed, even an empty signifier. Faced with this disturbance in the representational function of language, the analyst is led to interrogate, beyond the fantasmatic contents of remarks, the very status of language for these patients and thus the implications for the analyst's own interpretative discourse. An analysis of content goes hand in hand, it seems to me, with an analytical attentiveness which must be termed infra-semantic; it follows the disturbances of subjectivity in their most subtle aspects—in other words, in discourse itself, even in the function of words and sentences as signs and as elements of meaning. Through construction or condensation, through the economy of its own discourse and not only its content, interpretation itself is an encounter with the subject speaking to us which enables him to express himself at the point closest to his own destruction.

In what follows, I would like to concentrate on two aspects of borderline discourse: the *empty signifier,* which "treats words as things," and an *undecidable negation,* which "is unaware of repression." I will then add some comments on the role of different analytic interpretations in such instances.

The Empty Signifier

Whether it is perforated with silences or, on the contrary, over-saturated to the point of not tolerating the slightest interruption,

11. See, among other texts, the Winnicott chapter cited earlier.

the patient's "borderline" discourse gives the analyst the impression of something alogical, unstitched, and chaotic—despite its occasionally obsessive appearances—which is almost impossible to memorize. Once past this initial confusion ("but what was the patient talking about?"), the analyst is struck by a certain maniacal eroticization of speech, as if the patient were clinging to it, gulping it down, sucking on it, delighting in all the aspects of an oral eroticization and a narcissistic safety belt which this kind of noncommunicative, exhibitionistic, and fortifying use of speech entails. The analyst notices a tendency to play with signifiers: puns, portmanteau words, the condensation of signifiers, which are not always, not only, or sometimes not at all cultural acquisitions. Yet this manipulation of the signifier leaves the analyst, as well as the patient, at special moments—that is, moments of suffering—with a feeling of void, since it seems to be a discourse cut off from all *affect*.

In rereading Freud's initial, preanalytic text on aphasia and then appendix C of "The Unconscious" (*Standard Edition*, vol. 14), where we find Freud's own model of the *sign* and not the Saussurean signifier/signified distinction, we note first of all that perceptions (acoustic, tactile, visual, etc.) and different kinesthetic states are integrated within its matrix. We must rehabilitate this Freudian sign; the study of language—in linguistics or in psychoanalysis—can no longer do without it. Furthermore, if we ask who insures the liaison (cathexis), the psychic function of assembling all those word- and thing-presentations, the only answer is: the possibility of establishing a relation with a *third* party, with an "extra other" beyond the mother-child dyad. I must pass over the vast and very difficult question of the relation between *affect* and representation, or, more specifically, verbal representation. For the question that concerns us here is, How can we interpret this *emptying* of affect in the borderline signifier, this corporeal absence which hides suffering and which, I believe, produces a corollary semantic chaos in borderline discourse.

We might suppose a disintegration of the *"sign"* function in these patients. This would be only a *relative* disintegration because their discourse does function, sometimes with a semblance of socialization; nevertheless, it does represent a disintegration, which I will try to outline here.

A final reference to psychoanalytic theory will perhaps clarify this matter. In "Notes on Symbol Formation,"[12] Hanna Segal describes symbol formation as an activity of the ego which seeks to work out the anguish born of the ego-object relation. At first, within the "projective identification" between ego and Object, we find the constitution not of "symbols" (in the sense of "substitutes") but of *symbolic equivalences,* "symbolic equations" (which transpire as the "concrete thoughts" of schizophrenics). Only in a later stage—the so-called depressive stage—is the object perceived as total, thus differentiated from the ego and, through guilt, anguish, and mourning, re-created with *words* that are no longer equivalents but *repairers,* allowing the subject not to deny the loss of the object but rather to overcome this loss.

Borderline patients' attachment to the signifier, and the manipulation of meaning in which they indulge, could be viewed as dependent on these "symbolic equations" which are not yet signs in the sense that (1) the sign represents an object to a subject (Peirce), and (2) the signifier represents the subject for another signifier (Lacan). Yet it seems to me that the Klein-Segal explanation fails to account for the impression of *void,* which I described above, because it postulates from the beginning the existence of an *ego* and an *object.* On the contrary, everything indicates that when the infant is forming a "fusional dyad" with the genetrix, this differentiation is problematic, perhaps nonexistent, and this ego is entirely unstable. The *Object,* which is formed progressively through the processes of introjection and projection, is an *abject;*[13] the ego, in a similar fashion, cannot perceive completeness, but only void, hollowness, and injury.

I believe, therefore, that the idea of a happy fusional narcissism, and even the more dramatic notion of a projective identification, *fail to indicate, not the feeling of lack (tributary to castration), but*

12. *International Journal of Psycho-Analysis* 38 (1957): 391–97.

13. J. Kristeva, *Pouvoirs de l'horreur: Essai sur l'abjection* (Paris: Seuil, 1980). This work defines the intra-narcissistic relation between a not-yet Ego and an *abject,* a not-yet object, which prefigures the subject's later relation to the maternal object.

the feeling of emptiness which is at the root of the future ego's psychosomatic experiences. If "symbolic equations" exist, they move along two chasms—an *ab-ject* and an ego capable of becoming a hole, a void, empty of all kinesthetic experiences and affects. Such an ego overproduces a void *signifier,* empty of affect itself, and, through this emptiness, tries to fill the hole, to deny absence (infantile echolalia). The "good enough mother" is perhaps the one who hears this "void," supports it, plays with it, but fixates it as neither a void nor a perverse game; rather, she directs it toward the father—in other words, toward the Symbol. If depression follows, what prevents this depression from becoming endless melancholia? And what makes it (miraculously) a *sign?* It is the *Third,* the structuring function of the Third (father, psychotherapist, etc.). This echoing discourse, this echolalia, filling the dyad of these two emptiness-ridden terms, is directed toward the Third. "You talk to him about you/me; *he* gives meaning to our jubilant and emptying exchanges, we make a sign *to him.*" Only at this point in the dynamic process do the fragmented components of these "symbolic equations" become *condensed* into *signs* for the Other who is the Third; and on this basis, the mother can become an object, an Other; and not an Ab-ject.

The Undecidable Negation

Another particularity of borderline discourse strikes the analyst: the feeling that these patients can make statements of deep content (incestuous or murderous, for example) which would remain unconscious in the neurotic. This has led Fairbairn and Kernberg to postulate "a lack of repression" or a "problematic repression" in these patients.[14] Before responding to this hypothesis, I must note that the same patients often make indiscriminate use of antithetical couplets as if the negation (of certain highly charged contents) had no meaning. "She makes me live, no, she devitalizes me" or "She makes me neither live nor die" (a negation of two antithetical terms). One of my patients, for exam-

14. O. Kernberg, *Borderline Conditions and Pathological Narcissism* (New York: Jason Aronson, 1975).

ple, told me: "You're in front of me, no, you're behind, rather, you're *both* in front *and* behind. But how can that be? It reminds me of a swing glass in an amusement park." Several interpretations of this specular uncertainty come to mind, among them the following: if this negative sign makes no difference, if negation is no longer a sign, it is because the sign itself (which replaces an object for a subject) is emptied of affect and has no subjective meaning. These two phenomena (the uncertainty of negation and the release of condensation) are correlative.

This indifference to negation would seem to be related to the impression that these patients lack repression. But this would be a false impression, since it is hard to imagine how the acquisition of language or access to a certain type of socialization, which these patients possess, can be formed without repression. Instead, let us say that for the borderline, the repressed (similar here to what is denied) has *meaning* but no *signification*. I use Frege's distinction (*Sinn/Bedeutung*) here in a specific sense: *signification* is what subjective meaning has and this meaning fits into the subject's universe, incorporates his affects and experiences; it "means" something to him. If it "means" nothing to him, this indicates that no other has played the role of authenticator of his symbolic experience. Here again we see the absence of the paternal function through a chain reaction of symbolic deficiencies. In this case, the subject proffers contents that have an (absolute) *meaning* of repression but do not for him have the signification of the *repressed*.

Some Remarks on the Effects of the Analyst's Speech

Borderline discourse elicits a special transferential or countertransferential attitude which I shall not discuss here. I would note, however, in light of my remarks on some characteristics of borderline discourse in its dissolution of the "sign," the role that different analytic interpretations can play.

The analyst often feels called upon, especially in the beginning of a cure, to *construct relations,* to take up the bits of discursive chaos in order to indicate their relations (temporal, causal, etc.), or even simply to repeat these bits of discourse, thereby already ordering these chaotic themes. This kind of logical, even associative, task could give the impression that we work at constructing repression. More precisely, and in light of the "sign" function and its perturbations, these constructions serve to give the speech act a *signification* (for a subject—the analyst, the patient). This repetition or reordering by means of an interpretation that builds connections does not serve to reconstruct either a real or an imaginary biography. Instead, it reestablishes plus and minus signs and, subsequently, logical sequences and thus the very capacities of speech to enunciate exterior referential realities. And when this apparently logical, intellectual work is finished, affect is released into discourse.

Why does logic lead us to affect? It is because we have helped construct signs in relation to each other in their articulatory function. Some would say that this type of *constructive* interpretation functions as a holding pattern (Winnicott). I would suggest, rather, that in limiting oneself to the image of a holding pattern the analyst would be merely attempting to "repair" the patient's narcissistic image. On the other hand, if the analyst, in those moments, sees his own discourse as the *solder [soudure]* of the signifying function in its logical, syntactical dimension, he can avoid making the cure a sinking into dependence (a reduction of the subject to the egoic or imaginary dynamic of the mother-child relation). In short, constructive interpretation reestablishes signification and allows meaning to rediscover affect.

But what about "*condensed*" interpretations: metaphors, the play of signifiers, and so forth? "Condensation," says Freud in *Jokes and Their Relation to the Unconscious*, "[is] a process stretching over the whole course of events till the perceptual region is reached" (*Standard Edition*, vol. 8, p. 164). Thus, a condensed interpretation has a more erotic and more binding effect, but it also releases more instinctual drive and/or aggression; regardless of content, it is deeply inscribed in the transference dynamic. It activates all of the sign's components, but with no logico-constructive protection. It separates non-sense from the restrictions of meaning and colludes with the manic or narcissistic manipulation of the signifier in the borderline patient. It should be used prudently, in full knowledge that it inevitably entails a "maternal" type of transference, and the entire gamut of those desires and needs.

An example—one of my female patients who had a French mother and an unknown Vietnamese father. There were long sessions with no mention of the father, but in which the chaos of the unspoken, ellipses, and absence seemed, more than neurotic resistances, to be the true sufferings of "false selves." Then came the work of *constructing* upon this material, which finally evoked her interest in the mirror, where she concentrated on her clothes. She seemed to see only her clothes, nothing of her body. Interpretation: "It's as if clothes made you feel good about yourself" [*vous faisaient être bien dans votre peau*]. Then, after a silence, her first mention of a feeling of strangeness and, afterward, a fantasm of St. Christopher carrying the Infant Jesus on his shoulders. She doesn't know why this makes her feel so safe. Interpretation: "St. Christopher" sounds like the analyst's last name. Silence. "Yes, like when I was adopted by the Julien family." Silence. (Her adoptive family's name is completely different, but the signifier "Julien" suggests the analyst's first name.) "I don't know why I said that," then "I never thought it had anything to do with you. . . ."

At this point, it was crucial for the interpretation to emphasize *skin [peau]* (the border between outside and inside), birth, but also the *proper name*. The proper name is the signifier par excellence of Identity, in this case the analyst's identity as object of identification from whom the patient desires a second birth. But I particularly wanted to emphasize the *condensed interpretation* here. Coming at an opportune moment in the cure, it didn't pass unnoticed, nor did it appear unreal, or, if it did (was the mention of the Julien family a hallucination or a lie?), it prompted elaboration ("I never thought it had anything to do with you").

As closing note I want to comment on the place of these remarks in the current practice of interpretation. I am tempted to say that they have no place, since it is free-floating attentiveness, transference, and our own access to the unconscious which guide us in this obscure task of interpretation. To try to clarify it in a theoretical manner, as I have done here, is undoubtedly an attempt to utilize the anguish inherent in this obscure work—a temptation of mastery, of (obsessional) defense.

And yet, when the analyst who never ceases listening *also hears himself speak,* the mere act of keeping his ears open, not only to the content but also to the *dynamic of the sign*—some aspects of which I have outlined here—perhaps leads to subtler insights into the psyche. By subtle I mean *infra-semantic*—informed by the linguistic and psychic operations which constitute the sign's matrix and sign systems. In my view, this need is all the more acute when faced with discourses which proceed by stripping away if not disarticulating symbolic mechanisms.

This kind of "knowledge," provided that one can also disengage from it, can perhaps change our attitude toward our patients. For this ostensibly *formalist* attentiveness is perhaps an ethical guarantee: it should provide narcissistic traumas with a cure that can circumvent the pitfalls of "reparation" or fetishist-creativist solutions; and it can focus on the patient's own reintegration of the many and varied capacities of linguistic signs which constitute the only real identity.

Philosophy and Psychoanalytic Theory

4

Lacan and the Subject of Psychoanalysis

WILLIAM J. RICHARDSON

In the fall of 1981, readers of the sedate *New York Times* were startled by an unusually sensational headline—"Scholar Links Freud to Wife's Sister" (22 Nov. 1981, p. 26)—and the same news event subsequently supplied the occasion for a cover story in *Newsweek* (30 Nov. 1981, pp. 64–73). The story reported a lecture at New York University in which the historian Peter J. Swales postulated that in 1900 Freud had had a love affair with his wife's sister, Minna Bernays (who lived with them at the time), and arranged for an abortion for her in Italy that summer.

As reported, Swales based his argument in part on a rereading of an incident recounted in *The Psychopathology of Everyday Life* (1901, pp. 8–11). Freud there relates how he met on a train a well-educated young man of Jewish descent who complained bitterly of the anti-Semitism to which he was subjected and ended a fervent tirade by citing the line from Virgil's *Aeneid* in which Dido calls for vengeance upon Aeneas, "*Exoriare . . . .*" Or rather, he *tries* to cite the line but can't recall it exactly and asks Freud for help. Freud obliges by quoting the line exactly: "*Exoriar[e] ALIQUIS nostris ex ossibus ultor*" (*Aeneid* 4:625, literally: "Let someone (*aliquis*) arise from my bones as an avenger!"). Thereupon the young man, already familiar with Freud's claim that such words are not forgotten without reason, asks Freud to help him discover the reason for his forgetfulness here. Freud agrees and lays down the classic analytic rule to say "*candidly* and *uncritically*" whatever comes into mind when he focuses on the forgotten word.

The Edith Weigert Lecture, sponsored by the Forum on Psychiatry and the Humanities, Washington School of Psychiatry, October 16, 1981.

—

The young man begins by dividing the word into *a* and *liquis* and soon associates to *Reliquien* (relics), *liquefying, fluidity, fluid,* etc. There follows allusion to certain saints of the Church, such as Simon, Augustine, and Benedict, and the text continues:

"Now it's St. *Januarius* and the miracle of his blood that comes into my mind—my thoughts seem to me to be running on mechanically."

"Just a moment: St. *Januarius* and St. *Augustine* both have to do with the calendar. But won't you remind me about the miracle of his blood?"

"Surely you must have heard of that? They keep the blood of St. Januarius in a phial inside a church at Naples, and on a particular holy day it miraculously *liquefies.* The people attach great importance to this miracle and get very excited if it's delayed, as happened once at a time when the French were occupying the town. So the general in command—or have I got it wrong? was it Garibaldi?—took the reverend gentleman aside and gave him to understand, with an unmistakable gesture towards the soldiers posted outside, that he *hoped* the miracle would take place very soon. And in fact it did take place . . ."

"Well, go on. Why do you pause?"

"Well, something *has* come into my mind . . . but it's too intimate to pass on. . . .Besides, I don't see any connection, or any necessity for saying it."

"You can leave the connection to me. Of course I can't force you to talk about something that you find distasteful; but then you mustn't insist on learning from me how you came to forget your *aliquis.*"

"Really? Is that what you think? Well then, I've suddenly thought of a lady from whom I might easily hear a piece of news that would be very awkward for both of us."

"That her periods have stopped?"

"How could you guess that?"

"That's not difficult any longer; you've prepared the way sufficiently. Think of *the calendar saints, the blood that starts to flow on a particular day, the disturbance when the event fails to take*

*place, the open threats that the miracle must be vouchsafed, or
else. . . . In fact you've made use of the miracle of St. Januarius to manufacture a brilliant allusion to women's periods."* [1901, pp. 10–11]

So far the anecdote. Now Swales argued that the story as told is
really about Freud himself. If true, the allegation obviously
would throw new light on Freud the man. But would it vitiate the
insight that the alleged incident gives us into Freud's thought?
The claim here is that it would not. For even if this anecdote
turned out to be autobiographical and were shaped by Freud's
own special literary genre, what it tells us about the subject of
psychoanalysis remains of permanent value.

Of course, the term "subject of psychoanalysis" may be taken in
several ways. If we understand it to mean the "subject matter" of
psychoanalysis, then this is obviously the unconscious dimension
of human existence that Freud experienced in himself and confirmed in others (as allegedly here). But if we understand the
"subject" as one who undergoes the process of analysis, then the
subject of psychoanalysis would appear to be that individual
being in whom the unconscious is discerned—the "analysand," in
ordinary terminology, or in the case of Freud, Freud himself. But
who, or what, or where is that? And how are we to understand the
relationship between the unconscious as Freud discovered it and
the individual in whom it has its way? For Jacques Lacan, the
relationship between the two is a strange correlation, for he will
tell us that the unconscious of the subject is the subject of the
unconscious. Typical Lacanian enigma. What I propose in these
few pages is to try to disentangle it and explore some of its philosophical implications.

Lacan's fundamental thesis—this much, at least, is now a commonplace—is that Freud's epoch-making discovery of the unconscious was an insight into the way that language works: the unconscious is "structured like a language" (1977, p. 234/594).[1] By this,

---

1. In referring to texts of Lacan in English translation, I give first the page
reference to the English text, then the reference to the French text. Occasionally
these have been slightly emended. Where no published translation exists, texts
have been translated by the author.

Lacan means that the unconscious follows the same laws that language does, as these have been discerned by contemporary linguists following the lead of Ferdinand de Saussure long after Freud's own breakthrough.

Among the essentials of Saussure's discoveries was the distinction he made in terms of the classic conception of language as a system of signs; to Saussure the sign consists of a signifying component, the "signifier" (auditory image or speech sound), and the "signified" (the mental image corresponding to the verbal sound). Moreover, Saussure insisted on the arbitrary nature of the relation between signifier and signified; there is no intrinsically necessary bond between the sound image "horse" and the concept "horse"—*equus* or *cheval* would do as well. Furthermore, all signifiers, Saussure claimed, are related to each other according to the norm of any diacritical model. It was this linguistic model of a system of signifiers that served Lévi-Strauss so well in developing his conception of structural anthropology.

Lacan describes Saussure's conception in the form of an algorithm that sees the signifier as numerator of a fraction and the signified its denominator—the two separated by a bar that is meant now to indicate what for Saussure is the arbitrary nature of the relation between the two. But Lacan stresses the importance of this "bar," conceiving it as indeed a "barrier" to any one-to-one relationship between signifier and signified, insisting that any given signifier refers not to any corresponding signified but rather to another signifier in a sequence or "chain" of signifiers that Lacan describes as being like "rings of a necklace that is a ring in another necklace made of rings" (1977, p. 153/502). What is the meaning (signified) of such a chain? "We can say that it is in the chain of the signifiers that the meaning 'insists' but that none of its elements 'consists' in the signification of which it is at the moment capable. We are forced, then, to accept the notion of an incessant sliding of the signified under the signifier" (1977, pp. 153–54/502).

Concretely, what does this mean? In the conversation of Freud with his traveling companion (let's call him Simon) we can see how the forgotten word *aliquis,* taken as the starting point of Simon's

free association, soon leads to other signifiers, such as "liquefying," "liquid," "fluidity," "fluid," "relics," by a kind of proximity,
or rather contiguity, of one to the other (whether of sound, or
meaning, or etymology, etc.) along what the linguists call an "axis
of combination," which Lacan, following Jakobson and the old
rhetoricians (Jakobson, 1956, pp. 63–75), calls "metonymy." The
meaning of this chain does not "consist" in any one of these
elements but rather "insists" in the whole, where the "whole" may
be taken to be the entire interlude as described, whose meaning,
or rather whose "effect" of meaning, is discerned retroactively
when the discourse is punctuated by Freud's decisive question
about the cessation of periods. For our purposes, it suffices to
note that in this specimen of the psychoanalytic method:

1. the efficacious factor in the process is the spoken word;
2. Freud's ear is attuned principally to the sequence of Simon's
   signifiers, not to his emotional state;
3. in attempting to reveal the unconscious of the subject, Freud
   in effect discerns the subject of the unconscious.

What is the "subject of the unconscious"? At one point Lacan
actually calls it "unconscious subject" (1978, p. 218), meaning
unconscious *as* subject—the subject where the unconscious holds
sway. He speaks of the "truth discovered by Freud" as "the self's
(*soi*) radical ex-centricity to itself" (1977, p. 171/524). In other
words, there is in man a center of which he is not aware, by reason
of which he speaks without realizing it and therefore says more
than he knows (1972–73, p. 108). This center is ex-centric to the
center of his conscious life:

> The radical heteronomy that Freud's discovery shows gap-
> ing within man can never again be covered over without
> whatever is used to hide it being profoundly dishonest.
>
> Who, then, is this other to whom I am more attached than
> to myself, since, at the heart of my assent to my own identity it
> is still he who agitates me? [1977, p. 172/524]

In this ex-centric center there are "signifying mechanisms" by
reason of which it may legitimately be said to have "thoughts," to
"think" (1977, pp. 165–66/517). What is the nature of such

"mechanisms"? Here Lacan appeals to the perspective of Lévi-Strauss: before all human experience, whether individual or collective, the field in which this experience takes place is organized by certain predetermined relations.

> Nature furnishes, so as to speak, signifiers, and these signifiers organize in inaugural fashion [all] human relationships, supply [these relationships] with structures and shape them. . . . In our day, at an historical time when we are formed by a science which we can qualify as [specifically] human . . . , namely linguistics, whose model is the play of combinations (*jeu combinatoire*) operating spontaneously all alone in a pre-subjective manner—it is this structure that gives to the unconscious its status. [1964, pp. 20–21/23–24]

This is what Lévi-Strauss called the "symbolic order." Lacan accepts the term with a somewhat different emphasis, excluding any possible imaginary interpretation and insisting on its "law"-like quality. We shall return to this below.

Such, then, is the ex-centric center of the subject or "subject of the unconscious." Lacan occasionally describes it as a subject "without a head" (*acéphale*). "If there is an image which could represent for us the Freudian notion of the unconscious, it is indeed that of a subject without a head, of a subject which no longer has an *ego* . . . , de-centered with regard to the *ego,* which does not belong to the *ego.* And yet, it is a subject that speaks" (1954–55, p. 200). Subject without an ego, yet a subject that speaks! How is that possible?

Lacan takes as starting point for his conception of the ego an obvious ambiguity in Freud that became apparent in 1914–15 with "On Narcissism." There the ego, instead of being considered an agency, a substructure of the personality (of whatever kind), begins to be considered a love object. Freud speculates that:

- the ego is not present from the beginning but must be constituted by some "new psychical action";
- the ego appears as a unity relative to the anarchic, fragmentary functioning that characterizes autoerotism;
- under these circumstances, the ego presents itself as a love-object, just like external objects;

• thus the ego cannot be identified with the subject's internal world as a whole (see Laplanche and Pontalis, 1967, p. 137).

We are all aware of the vagaries of the notion of "ego" in Freud in other texts, especially after 1920, which gave warrant to ego psychologists such as Hartmann, Kris, and Loewenstein to elaborate the notion of the ego as mediator between id, superego, and "reality"—agent of synthesis for the entire personality. For Lacan, however, the 1914 notion of the ego as love-object is decisive. His own interpretation of the conception was first proposed at the Marienbad International Congress of Psychoanalysis in 1936. Basing his case on data taken from child psychology concerning the infant's behavior when first confronted with his own reflection in a mirror, and also on data taken from animal ethology indicating how certain maturational processes are possible only after visual perception of the species counterpart, Lacan argues that sometime between the ages of six and eighteen months the infant, fragmented by the turmoil of its anarchic urges, perceives "with a flutter of jubilation" a reflection of itself, whether in a counterpart or in a mirror, as a form (Gestalt) by which it anticipates a bodily unity still to be achieved in fact, and with which it identifies. This reflected, therefore alienated image becomes the ideal of eventual unity, the basis for all subsequent identification, and its citadel of defense (1977, pp. 1–7).

The infant, then, caught up in identification with its mirror image, is locked into a bipolar image-world—that is, in the register of what Lacan calls the imaginary. And the ego for Lacan never ceases to be anything more than an object—"an object (to be sure) that fulfills a certain function" (1954–55, p. 60)—the first task of which is to supply a focus of unity to the subject and in that way to determine on a certain level the "structuration" of the subject (1954–55, p. 68). As an analogue, Lacan suggests that we try to imagine an adult paralytic before a mirror, unable to move alone except in the most awkwardly cumbersome manner. What controls his movement is the mirror image (his "ego"), which stares back at him blindly and fascinates him. Sole source of his coordinated—that is, unified—movement, it is the image that "carries" him about like a slave (1954–55, pp. 66–68).

The ego, then, is not the subject but the alienated image of the subject—more precisely, of the subject-to-be. How does the subject emerge in the young organism? We have some idea of this from the way Lacan interprets Freud's famous anecdote of his grandchild, who, with the "oh" and *da*" of the *fort-da* ("away"-"here") experience of making a toy reel disappear and return, plays the game of making his mother disappear and return (1920, pp. 14–15). What is striking in this for Lacan is not the fact that by this game of substituting a toy reel for his mother the child learns to control his libidinal urges, but rather that through the exercise of these primitive phonemes the child discovers the marvelous secret that what is absent can be rendered present through signifiers, for he thereby enters into the symbolic order.

How Lacan weaves this initial experience of language into the fabric of the oedipal drama need not concern us here. Rather, let us ask ourselves how the subject can say "I" independently of his fascination with his own imaginary ego. In ordinary discourse, the "I" of the speaker may be understood in at least two different senses: (1) as the "I" of the formulated statement that serves as "subject" of all affirmations in the first person—for example, Simon's remark: "I should be very curious to learn how I came to forget the indefinite pronoun *'aliquis.'* " This is the "I" of conscious discourse. (2) As the "I" of the speaker that recedes from the statement in the very act of making it—the articulating "I" as opposed to the articulated "I"—the "I" who slips behind the spoken word, or underneath the succession of signifiers, and is, as it were, suspended from them (e.g., Simon as the "I"—victim of forgetting). This is the "I" who is subject to the *un*conscious discourse. For Lacan, the subject is "not the living substrate . . . nor any sort of substance . . . nor any being of knowledge . . . nor even the logos becoming incarnate somewhere, but the Cartesian subject which appears at the moment when doubt is recognized as certitude" (1964, p. 126/116, slightly emended). *This* is the subject that is ex-centrically centered, that is agitated by the Other in its slips, its parapraxia, its forgetfulness, its dreams.

The "Cartesian subject"! As Lacan sees it, there would have been no Freud had there been no Descartes, for the unconscious

Freud discovered is the unconscious of this kind of subject. We recall Descartes's endeavor: to find an unshakable foundation for truth, certified truth—that is, truth carrying within it its own guarantee, truth in the sense of "certitude." His methodic doubt ended with the famous *cogito*, to the effect that the very doubting yielded at least one certitude: "I, while thinking, am." There is, of course, a self-transparency discerned in the immediate reflection that constitutes this experience and has come to be associated with consciousness, and it was this self-aware certitude that became itself the foundation—unshakable because self-validating— of all truth. As foundation, it was by that very fact the underlying stratum (the Greeks would have said *hypokeimenon*, the Latins *subjectum*) or "subject" of all truth. Of course, it was easy to interpret this conscious, self-conscious, ego-preoccupied subject as *subsistens, substans:* a subsistent self-contained subject—as many obviously did.

But the fact remains that the subject which says "I think, I am" *says* it. It is not simply a self-conscious, ego-oriented subject but a *speaking* one, and, blinded by the luminous transparency of its own presence to itself, this subject discerned by Descartes is unaware of the opaqueness of the signifying (system) that determined it as it spoke. It was here that Freud would discover in it a de-centered center.

The subject of psychoanalysis, then, is the Cartesian subject which appears at the moment when doubt is recognized as certitude. It appears in and as the articulating of the "thinking-am." The French linguist Emile Benveniste has pointed out that personal pronouns in general and the "I" in particular do not refer either to a concept or to an individual discourse in which they are pronounced and appear to designate the speaker. It is a term that can be identified only in what has been called an instance of discourse and has no other reference than a momentary (*actuelle*) one. The reality to which it refers is the reality of the discourse. Others speak of it as a "shifter," shifting its meaning according to context. "It is in the instance of the discourse in which *I* designates the speaker that the latter is articulated as a subject. It is, then, literally true that the foundation of subjectivity is in the exercise of language" (Benveniste, 1972, pp. 261–62, my translation), even though the speaker may be using the third person.

Lacan draws rigorous consequences from this fact. If "the foundation of subjectivity is in the exercise of language," and if "I" can be identified only in terms of the actual moment of the discourse, then the speaking subject *as such* is sustained by the discourse *as such*—that is, by the chain of signifiers—and we arrive at some understanding of what Lacan means by saying that the subject must be defined as "the effect of the signifier." And when he contends that although a sign represents indeed something for someone, a signifier is that which "represents a subject for another signifier" (1966, p. 840), we infer that the subject (e.g., Simon) for Lacan is essentially what is represented by the congeries of its signifiers. It is the signifier, then, that constitutes the subject—and more profoundly than any element that could be called "psychological" (1964, p. 142/130). "The displacement of the signifier determines the subjects in their acts, in their destiny, in their refusals, in their blindnesses, in their end and in their fate, their innate gifts and social acquisitions notwithstanding, without regard for character and sex. . . . Willingly or not, everything that might be considered the stuff of psychology, kit and caboodle, will follow the path of the signifier" (1955, p. 60/30).

What more can be said of this "order of signifiers"? First of all that it *is* an order, an arrangement of relationships that has enough stability and firmness to be called a "law." Lacan will even call it *the* Law, indeed the Law of *the* Father, however that fatherhood is to be conceived. Moreover, the pattern of relationships has been woven into the entire fabric of human history to which the infant now falls heir as he becomes "subject to," and thereby made a subject of (*assujetissement*), this Law. This fabric includes the cultural myths of his race, his ethnic style, his social traditions, the patricularity of his ancestral lineage, the personal and social milieu of his immediate family (e.g., the full scope of Simon's Jewishness from before the birth of Abraham down to his own circumcision)—in short, the universal "discourse" that has preceded him and into which he has been born.

But the pattern of relationships is more than just the sedimentation of cultural and personal history. Lacan refers to it as a "circuit" into which the subject is "integrated" (1954–55, p. 112)—one gets the image of a kind of cosmic electrical system. This system is a network that is governed by its own laws, which the linguists call "synchrony" (see 1964, pp. 26/28, 188/172) and Lacan conceives to be laws of a combinatory system; a system that functions through operative principles governing possible combinations of relationships of signifiers that, when all is said and done, are ultimately reducible to the yes/no, plus/minus options of the simplest computer system, a series of sluice gates that permit or do not permit the current to pass according to whether they are or are not open. "Every machine can be reduced to a series of relays that are simply a [matter of] *plus* and *minus*. Everything in the symbolic order can be represented with the help of such a succession" (1954–55, p. 218). It is in the understanding of such a combinatory system that Lacan sees the contribution of structural linguistics. At any rate, it is this lottery of combinations (*jeu combinatoire*) that, when the unconscious subject intrudes into conscious discourse (as in the forgetting of *aliquis*), accounts for the unpredictability (the surprise character and discontinuity [1964, p. 25/27]) of these intrusions.

Now, this "order of signifiers" in all its complexity (as symbolic order, as Law of the Father, as concrete discourse, as universal circuit, as *jeu combinatoire*, and eventually as locus of truth) Lacan designates as "the Other," that is, as pure alterity as such. The integration of the individual into the Other constitutes the "subject-ifying" of the subject, its radical division ("splitting"). "The subject is born insofar as in the field of the Other the signifier emerges. But by this very fact, what formerly was nothing but [a] subject-to-come [*sujet à venir*] congeals in [a] signifier" (1964, p. 199/181, slightly emended). To signalize this in writing, Lacan designates the subject by a capital "S," but then puts a bar through it to indicate its radical division ($): "We symbolize by the barred subject ($) the subject insofar as [it is] constituted as subsequent to its relation to [*second par rapport au*] the signifier" (1964, p. 141/129, slightly emended). It is in this radical cleavage of the subject through insertion into the Other that Lacan situates "primary repression" and, indeed, the essential nature of castration. Understood in all rigor, then, the subject as such—for example Simon as subject—does not exist before the submersion into the order of signifiers, nor outside of that order, but only within it, as represented and sustained by the sequence of signifiers of which it is in continual want if it is to remain a subject.

Now, inasmuch as the subject is suspended from the sequence of signifiers, one may say that it recedes behind each of the signifiers that sustains it. This receding Lacan refers to as the "fading" of the subject behind the signifier, and in another context, capitalizing on a term introduced by Ernest Jones to designate a putative fear that sexual desire may disappear, the *a-phanisis* (from the Greek, *a-phaino*, meaning "dis-appear")—that is, the dis-appearing of the subject behind the signifier (1964, pp. 207–29, 189–210). Inversely, Lacan speaks of the "fluctuating" (*battement*) or "vacillating" way in which the unconscious vanishes as soon as it appears—always elusively, always evasively—in its irruptions into consciousness (1964, pp. 28/29, 32/33), as in any slip of the tongue (e.g., after entrapping *aliquis*, it does not stay around to take a bow).

Such, then, is the subject of the unconscious—a true subject insofar as, ex-centric to the ego, it can speak and infiltrate the articulating "I" (1954–55, p. 16). It is increasingly clear, however, that the unconscious as subject is by no means coincident with the human individual, or with the animal organism that it inhabits. "There is an animal that finds itself speaking and for whom it comes to pass that by dwelling in the signifying [system] it is subject to (*en*) [of?] [that system]" (1972–73, p. 81). Such is the sense that Lacan gives to the famous phrase of Rimbaud: "I is another" (*je est un autre*) (1954–55, p. 17). This other center transcends the individual the way a numerical system "transcends" the individuals it enumerates.

> What is important for us is to see here [in the order of signifiers] the level on which, before all formation of the subject . . . that thinks [and] is situated on that level, there is a counting [*ça compte*], there is a count, and in this count the count-er already is. It is only afterwards that the subject has

[the task of] recognizing itself . . . as count-er . . . [as in the case of] the little [boy] who says: "I have three brothers: Paul, Ernest and myself." [1964, p. 20/24]

Subject to the other, whether this be understood as the symbolic order as such, or as the chain of signifiers that have marked a personal history, or the combinatory game with its "presubjective" spontaneity, the human subject is no "master in its own house." The result is a determinism that for Lacan is clear and unequivocal:

This discourse . . . is the discourse of the circuit in which I am integrated. I am one of its links. It is the discourse of my father, for example, insofar as my father has committed faults that I am absolutely condemned to reproduce. [1954–55, p. 112]

Naturally, the subject can pass its whole life without attending to what is at stake. That is even what happens most commonly. Analysis is made so that he may attend to it, so that he may understand in what circle (*rond*) of the discourse he is caught up and in what other circle he has to enter. [1954–55, p. 123]

Or, to change the metaphor: "The game is already played, the dice are already cast . . . with this exception, that we may take them in hand again and cast them once more. . . . Don't you find something ridiculous and laughable in the fact that the dice are [already] cast?" (1954–55, p. 256).

Given all this, we can understand why and how Lacan insists on reinterpreting Freud's famous dictum: *Wo es war soll ich werden* (1933, p. 80). The sense is obviously not: "Where id was, there shall ego be," where ego would be understood as an agency that adapts libidinal urges to the demands of superego and "reality." Rather, the sense must be: "Where It [i.e., the network of signifiers that constitutes the Other] was, I-as-articulator [i.e., the subject as divided by reason of its ex-centric center] must come to be, that is, must realize my relation to, place within, that network. How? "It is by returning, by going back, by crossing one's [own] path" (1964, p. 45/45) again and again that the network comes to light. Such, indeed, is the task of psychoanalysis.

All this may seem abstruse and disembodied. Let us try to give it more flesh and blood by seeing how this subject functions in a dream. It may be helpful to sketch Lacan's reexamination of Freud's master dream analysis that served as model for all the rest—the "dream of dreams," as Lacan calls it, about the injection of Irma (1900, pp. 106–121). In his seminar "The Ego in the Theory of Freud and in the Technique of Psychoanalysis" (1954–55), Lacan turns to this dream à propos of the notion of "regression," and because of Erik Erikson's classic reinterpretation of that dream (1954), Lacan takes Erikson as his whipping boy. An avowed ego-psychologist, Erikson represents for Lacan the "culturalist" tendency in psychoanalysis that would accent what in any given case pertains to the "cultural" (for Erikson, "psychosocial") context into which he is plunged (1954–55, p. 179). Lacan is referring, of course, to Erikson's conception of the different stages of the "life cycle," according to which he postulates "tentative criteria for the ego's relative success in synthesizing, at crucial stages, the timetable of the organism and the representative demands which societies universally, if in different ways, provide for these stages" (1954, p. 35). The reader is no doubt familiar with the way Erikson differentiates these stages: successive periods of development characterized, for example, by issues of basic trust/mistrust (infancy), autonomy/shame-doubt (early childhood), initiative/guilt (oedipal stage), workmanship/inferiority (school age), identity/role diffusion (adolescence), intimacy/isolation (young adulthood), generativity/ stagnation (middle age) ("generativity" being the desire in every man to leave some lasting progeny for posterity). Since the Irma dream occurs during a lonely creative crisis when the dreamer is thirty-nine years old, it must be understood, Erikson claims, in conjunction with Freud's midlife crisis of generativity (1954, pp. 35–36).

Lacan, however, will have none of it. "If this point of view is true, we must abandon the notion that I claim to be in the essence of the Freudian discovery, the decentering of the subject with regard to the ego. . . .If it is true, everything I say is false" (1954–55, p. 179).

The dream, of course, is an old chestnut: Irma was one of Freud's hysterical patients whose treatment had gone fairly well, though some symptoms still remained. Just before interrupting for the summer, Freud made a suggestion to Irma that she refused to accept, so they parted in disagreement. During the summer a mutual acquaintance and younger medical colleague of Freud's, Otto, visited him. Asked about Irma, Otto replied, "She's better, but not quite well." Freud took this remark as reproof, became annoyed without saying so, wrote out the case history that evening to justify himself to himself, and later had the following dream:

> A large hall—numerous guests, whom we were receiving.—Among them was Irma. I at once took her on one side, as though to answer her letter and to reproach her for not having accepted my "solution" yet. I said to her: "If you still get pains, it's really only your fault." She replied: "If you only knew what pains I've got now in my throat and stomach and abdomen—it's choking me"—I was alarmed and looked at her. She looked pale and puffy. I thought to myself that after all I must be missing some organic trouble. I took her to the window and looked down her throat, and she showed signs of recalcitrance, like women with artificial dentures. I thought to myself that there was really no need for her to do that.—She then opened her mouth properly and on the right I found a big white patch; at another place I saw extensive whitish grey scabs upon some remarkable curly structures which were evidently modelled on the turbinal bones of the nose.—I at once called in Dr. M., and he repeated the examination and confirmed it. . . . Dr. M. looked quite different from usual; he was very pale, he walked with a limp and his chin was clean-shaven. . . . My friend Otto was now standing beside her as well, and my friend Leopold was percussing her through her bodice and saying: "She has a dull area low down on the left." He also indicated that a portion of the skin

on the left shoulder was infiltrated. (I noticed this, just as he did, in spite of her dress.) . . . M. said: "There's no doubt it's an infection, but no matter; dysentery will supervene and the toxin will be eliminated." . . . We were directly aware, too, of the origin of the infection. Not long before, when she was feeling unwell, my friend Otto had given her an injection of a preparation of propyl, propyls . . . propionic acid . . . trimethylamin (and I saw before me the formula for this printed in heavy type). . . . Injections of that sort ought not to be made so thoughtlessly. . . . And probably the syringe had not been clean. [1900–01, p. 107]

The gist of the dream, then, is clear: Irma has an infected throat; the reason is that Otto had given her an injection of trimethylamin with a dirty syringe.

Freud's own interpretation is, of course, classic:

The conclusion of the dream . . . was that I was not responsible for the persistence of Irma's pains, but that Otto was. . . . The dream acquitted me of the responsibility for Irma's condition by showing that it was due to other factors—it produced a whole series of reasons. The dream represented a particular state of affairs as I should have wished it to be. *Thus its content was the fulfilment of a wish and its motive was a wish.* [1900–01, pp. 118–19; Freud's italics]

Neither Erikson nor Lacan presumes to challenge Freud's interpretation of the dream in terms of wish fulfillment. Each reexamines the dream only in order to expand that interpretation. Both agree that the wish fulfilled by the dream should by Freud's criteria be called "preconscious" rather than "unconscious," and Lacan asks what it reveals, then, about the unconscious, since Freud seems to imply that it does reveal something in this regard (1954–55, p. 183). Both agree that the dream falls into two major parts, the first culminating in Freud's looking down Irma's throat, the second marked by Freud's appeal to others for help and the ultimate blaming of Otto. Both agree that Freud's looking into Irma's throat confronts him with the terrors of exploring (as he had been doing) the unknown. Both agree, finally, that the dream offers a solution to one tantalizing question that dominated at the time his explorations into the nature of mental illness—that is, about the meaning of dreams. In other words, both seem to admit that the dream was dreamed in order to be analyzed.

Erikson sees the matter this way:

> The doctor's growing sense of harboring a discovery apt to *generate new thought* had been challenged the night before. . . . At first, he vigorously and angrily asserts his most experienced use of one of the ego's basic functions: he examines, localizes, diagnoses. Such *investigation in isolation . . .* is one of the cornerstones of this dreamer's sense of *Inner Identity.* What he succeeds in focusing on, however, is a terrifying discovery which stares at him like the head of the Medusa. At this point, one feels, a dreamer with less flexible defenses might have awakened in terror over what he saw in the gaping cavity. Our dreamer's ego, however, makes the compromise of abandoning its positions and yet maintaining them. Abandoning independent observation, the dreamer gives in to a *diffusion of roles:* is he doctor or patient, leader or follower, benefactor or culprit, seer or fumbler? He admits to the possibility of his *inferiority in workmanship* and urgently appeals to "teacher" and to "teacher's pets." He thus forfeits his right to vigorous *male initiative* and guiltily surrenders to the inverted solution of the oedipal conflict, for a fleeting moment even becoming the feminine object for the superior males' inspection and percussion; and he denies his sense of stubborn *autonomy,* letting *doubt* lead him back to the earliest infantile security: childlike *trust. . . .*
>
> The ego, by letting itself return to sources of security once available to the dreamer as a child, may help him to dream well and to sustain sleep, while promising revengeful comeback in a new day. [1954, pp. 36–37]

Lacan sees it otherwise. Rejecting Erikson's conception of the ego, he obviously rejects as well his interpretation of the dream as "regression in the service of the ego,"[2] and claims that it violates the spirit of Freudian theory:

> For indeed if the *ego* is this succession of emergences . . . , if this double visage . . . of realisations and modes of non-real-isation constitutes its type, one has trouble seeing how to reconcile it with what Freud says in one or two thousand places in his writings, [namely], that the ego (*moi*) is the sum of identifications of the subject, with all that that can involve of the radically contingent. If I may express it by an image, the ego (*moi*) is like putting on top of one another different overcoats borrowed from what I call the bric-à-brac of its store of accessories. [1954–55, pp. 186–87]

What interpretation does he propose instead? Lacan agrees completely with Erikson's remark that after the horrifying look down Irma's oral cavity one would expect the dreamer to awaken. If he did not, the reason is not that the ego regressed to an earlier stage of development but rather that there was a "spectral decomposition" of the function of the ego—imaginary, of course—into a series of identifications which, useful in their time, has crystallized for the subject essential orientations at significant historical moments of his life (1954–55, p. 197). In this "destructuring" of the ego, the relations of the subject change completely. It becomes something totally different; there is no longer a Freud, but a multiplicity of figures (Dr. M., Otto, Leopold, etc.) representing Freud, as if the subject now had many heads, or rather, no head at all, egoless—"and yet a subject who speaks, for it is he who forces the personages who are in the dream to maintain their nonsensical discourse" and eventually articulates the key word, "trimethylamin" (1954–55, p. 200).

In the second part of the dream, then, as Lacan sees it, Freud's ego has been decomposed, and the dreamer emerges under the guise of Dr. M., Otto, and Leopold. But Freud's associations and subsequent references suggest other clusters of three: for exam-

2. The formula is from Kris (1950), but Erikson refers to it in a note (1954, p. 35), apparently with approval.

ple, three women in Freud's life, three paternal figures (Dr. M., Freud's older brother, Emmanuel, and Fleischl, the man who accidentally poisoned himself with cocaine), three peer figures (Otto, Leopold, Fliess). For our purposes the important element here is the number 3, the "mystic trio" as Lacan calls it. That seems to have had a special fascination for Freud.[3] In all this Lacan stresses: (1) the specifically triadic nature of the relationships involved; and (2) the gist of the conversation, ridiculous in itself, that expresses the dreamer's fundamental concern at the moment: What is the nature of mental illness? More specifically, what is the meaning of dreams?

In this maelstrom (of course, I abbreviate) there appears the word "trimethylamin," the dreamer adding, "and I saw before me the formula for this printed in heavy type." For Lacan, this is the culminating moment of the dream. "Trimethylamin" is a substituted ammonia containing three methyl groups: $N(CH_3)_3$. In other words, it is a chemical compound containing one atom of nitrogen bonded to three atoms of carbon, each of which in turn is bonded to three atoms of hydrogen. Visually speaking, it is a system of triads, to each element of which is linked a subtriad, all stemming from one central point (N), like a Christmas tree laid on its side. Lacan diagrams it thus:

```
                  /H
            C <--H
          /       \H
         /          /H
   N----C <-----H
         \          \H
          \          /H
            C <--H
                  \H
```

Chemists may be more familiar with another type of diagram:

---

3. For example, "The Theme of the Three Caskets" (1913). Forrester (1980, pp. 188–93) has a useful comment on the issue.

$$\begin{array}{c}
\text{H}\diagdown \\
\text{H}\!\rightarrow\!\text{C}\!-\!\text{N} \\
\text{H}\diagup
\end{array}
\begin{array}{c}
\text{C}\!\!\overset{\displaystyle\text{H}}{\underset{\displaystyle\text{H}}{\longleftarrow}}\!\text{H} \\[1ex]
\text{C}\!\!\overset{\displaystyle\text{H}}{\underset{\displaystyle\text{H}}{\longleftarrow}}\!\text{H}
\end{array}$$

In any case, the diagram expresses in the pure form of a chemical formula the triadic structures just mentioned. *This* dream at least has a clear symbolic structure that can be expressed in the rigor of a scientific formula and sketched in the diagram of a chemical structure; in this guise there is an answer to the question that Freud himself had been posing for months as to whether dreams in general have a meaning—that is a symbolic structure (obviously they do!); the function of the word "trimethylamin" as distinct from the visual presentation of the formula is precisely to bring the symbolic structure into a word. In effect, "this word doesn't mean anything except that it is a word" (1954–55, p. 202)—hence, the function of the symbolic order is precisely to come into word. "We can trace [the message of the dream for Freud] according to the Islamic formula, 'There is no other God than God,' [by saying that] there is no other word, no other solution to your problem [about the meaning of dreams] than the word" (1954–55, p. 190).

Notice, however, that this response does not emerge from Freud as an ego, but rather as from a subject without a head, from the Other, from that which is in the subject and "is both of the subject and not of the subject, [i.e.,] the unconscious" (1954–55, p. 191). Lacan concludes:

> When [Freud] interprets this dream, it is to us that he speaks . . . through the intermediary of the dream. . . . "I am he [Freud seems to say] who wants to be pardoned for having dared to begin to heal those persons whom up to now no one wanted to understand and whom one was forbidden to heal. I am he who wants to be pardoned for that. I am he who wants not to be guilty of it, for to transgress a limit imposed on human activity up to that time is always to be

guilty. I want not to be such a one. In place of me there are all the rest. I am there only as the representative of this vast, vague movement which is the search for truth, where I am effaced. I am no longer anything. My ambition has been greater than I. The syringe was dirty no doubt. And precisely in the measure that I desired too much, that I participated in this action, where I wanted to be the creator, I am not the creator. The creator is someone greater than I. It is my unconscious. It is this word that speaks in me, beyond me."
[1954–55, p. 203]

"That's the meaning of the dream," says Lacan. And that is Lacan's understanding of the unconscious as subject, the subject without a head.

But is that all that can be said? If the unconscious is headless, and if the speaking subject is no more than what is represented by a signifier for another signifier and, therefore, is in constant want of successive signifiers to be and to remain a subject, then who is Sigmund Freud the individual? What gives unity to this unique and dauntless explorer of the unknown who may have proven to be quite ordinary during the summer of 1900? For that matter, how explain the unity—I don't speak of totality—of a Jacques Lacan, whose turbulent career managed to preserve its equilibrium by means of a single gyroscope—that is, by his self-proclaimed fidelity to himself? Lacan himself, to be sure, scoffs at the question of unity in terms of the unconscious: "The one introduced by the experience of the unconscious is the one of the split . . . of rupture" (1964, p. 26/28). In terms of the articulating "I," he tells us:

> My experience has shown me that the principal characteristic of my own human life and, I am sure, that of the people who are here . . . is that life is something which goes, as we say in French, *à la dérive*. Life goes down the river, from time to time touching a bank, staying for a while here and there, without understanding anything—it is the principle of analysis that nobody understands anything of what happens. The idea of the unifying unity of the human condition has always had on me the effect of a scandalous lie. [1970, p. 190]

Be that as it may, I suggest that more can and must be said. For Descartes's conception of himself as a subject is not the last word on the nature of man. And even Freud, à propos of the Irma dream, suggests a depth in human beings beyond their ken. "There is at least one spot in every dream at which it is unplumbable—a navel, as it were, that is its point of contact with the unknown" (1900–01, p. 111n). Lacan, commenting, describes this as a point "ungraspable in the phenomenon, the point where there arises the relation of the subject to the symbolic. What I call Being is this last word, which is not accessible to us, certainly, in the scientific stance [*position*] but the direction of which is indicated in the phenomena of our experience" (1954–55, p. 130). Is it possible to think of this "unknown," "ungraspable" depth, then, as the Being of the subject? If so, then the subject's *want* of signifiers in order to remain a subject may be simply its want-to-be, its being-in-want. But "want-to-be" (*manque à être*) is Lacan's formula for *desire*.

To pose the question about the unity of the "who" engaged in the psychoanalytic process, precisely in terms of the unique human being who bears a name, we might explore the nature of desire. This would suggest that we follow either of two paths—eventually, no doubt, both. The first would be to interrogate the subject in its Being—that is, as process rather than as substance or subject (*hypokeimenon*) whose task is to be (and, therefore, is in want of being), process that as such does not say "I" but precedes the saying and remains always capable of it. There are several paradigms that we could explore. One would be that of Heidegger, for whom *Dasein* is a self that is precisely *not* a Cartesian subject but Being-in-the-World that is some*one* (always *je meines* [1927, p. 42]) that can and eventually *does* say "I." The unity of this self, we know, is not grounded in the reflection of a body image but in the unity of the triple ecstases of time. Another paradigm might be that of the later Merleau-Ponty, for whom subjectivity emerges out of the dehiscence of Being, of which it serves as a place of "openness." Temporality, then, would be a continued advent of Being. This would suggest a fresh and deeper meaning of the earlier formula of the *Phenomenology of Percep-*

tion, "The explosion or dehiscence of the present towards a future is the archetype of the relationship of self to self" (1945, p. 426) that makes self-awareness (consciousness) in the subject possible. Language plays a role of immense importance in both of these conceptions.

A second approach would be to explore the subject precisely in terms of its want-to-be, its primordial lack—that is, its desire. But to do justice to Lacan's understanding of desire, we would have to examine what S. Leclaire calls (1981, p. 167) "the discovery of Lacan"—the function of that object that "causes" desire, designated by the small letter "a" to suggest alterity in its purest form—and anonymity, too. It is this *objet a* that would give unity, then, to what some have even referred to as a "quasi-*Dasein*"—whatever that might mean. The philosophical paradigm here would be, of course, the dialectic of desire in Hegel, though Heidegger would also have a word to say about the "desire of the Other." This theme is explored in the following chapter.

Let us conclude for the present with one text of Lacan that is singularly inconclusive, but useful to close with because of what it opens up. "A certificate tells me that I was born," he said in the preface to an English translation. "[But] I repudiate that certificate. For I am not a poet but a poem. A poem that is being written, even if it looks like a subject" (1964, p. viii). The question now becomes: How can a poem be a some*one* who bears a name—even if it looks like a subject?

REFERENCES

Benveniste, E. *Problèmes de la linguistique générale.* Paris: Gallimard, 1972.

Erikson, E. H. "The Dream Specimen of Psychoanalysis." *Journal of the American Psychoanalytic Association* 2 (1954): 5–56.

Forrester, J. *Language and the Origins of Psychoanalysis.* New York: Columbia University Press, 1980.

Freud, S. *Standard Edition of the Complete Psychological Works.* London: Hogarth, 1953–74.

The Interpretation of Dreams (1900–01), vols. 4, 5.

The Psychopathology of Everyday Life (1901), vol. 6.

"The Theme of the Three Caskets" (1913), vol. 12.
"On Narcissism. An Introduction" (1914), vol. 14.
Beyond the Pleasure Principle (1920), vol. 18.
New Introductory Lectures on Psycho-Analysis (1933), vol. 22.
Gelman, D., and Hager, M. "Finding the Hidden Freud." *Newsweek,* 30 November 1981, pp. 64–73.
Heidegger, M. *Being and Time* (1927). Translated by J. Macquarrie and E. Robinson. New York: Harper & Row, 1962.
Jakobson, R. "Two Aspects of Language and Two Types of Aphasic Disturbances." In R. Jakobson and M. Halle, *Fundamental of Language.* The Hague: Mouton, 1956.
Kris, E. "On Preconscious Mental Process." *Psychoanalytic Quarterly* 19 (1950): 540–60.
Lacan, J.
Le Séminaire: Livre I. Les écrits techniques de Freud (1953–54). Paris: Seuil, 1975.
Le Séminaire: Livre II. Le moi dans la théorie de Freud et dans la technique de la psychanalyse (1954–55). Paris: Seuil, 1978.
"The Seminar on 'The Purloined Letter'" (1955). Translated by J. Mehlman. *French Freud: Structural Studies in Psychoanalysis, Yale French Studies* 48 (1972).
The Four Fundamental Concepts of Psycho-Analysis (1964). Translated by A. Sheridan. New York: Norton, 1978.
Écrits: A Selection (1966). Translated by A. Sheridan: New York: Norton, 1977.
"Of Structure as an Inmixing of Otherness Prerequisite to Any Subject Whatsoever" (1970). In R. Macksey and E. Donato, eds., *The Structuralist Controversy.* Baltimore: Johns Hopkins University Press, 1972.
Le Séminaire: Livre XX. Encore (1972–73). Paris: Seuil, 1975.
Laplanche, J., and Pontalis, J.-B. *The Language of Psychoanalysis* (1967). Translated by D. Nicholson-Smith. New York: Norton, 1973.
Leclaire, S. *Rompre les charmes. Receuil pour des enchantés de la psychanalyse.* Paris: Intereditions, 1981.
Merleau-Ponty, M. *Phenomenology of Perception* (1945). Translated by C. Smith. London: Routledge and Kegan Paul, 1962.
Virgilius Maro, Publius. *Opera, II.* Hildesheim: Olins, 1968.

5

Hegel, Heidegger, Lacan:
The Dialectic of Desire

EDWARD S. CASEY AND J. MELVIN WOODY

Psychoanalysis is constantly tempted by reductionism. That temptation stems from the desire to establish psychology on a genuinely "scientific" basis and to attain the rigor of the natural sciences by explaining the human in terms of the nonhuman. If all dimensions of human mental life could be translated into the terms of the sciences of nature, the recognizably human would be *reduced* to something already explained by "real" sciences such as physics and biology. The danger, of course, is that we may no longer recognize ourselves in the image which results—that the peculiarly human will somehow be lost in the reducing glass.

Freud himself was an eloquent spokesman for such a strategy. The opening of his "Project for a Scientific Psychology" provides a classic statement of this reductionist program:

> The intention [of this project] is to furnish a psychology that shall be a natural science: that is, to represent psychical processes as quantitatively determinate states of specifiable material particles, thus making those processes perspicuous and free from contradiction. Two principal ideas are involved: (1) What distinguishes activity from rest is to be regarded as Q [quantity], subject to the general laws of motion. (2) The neurones are to be taken as the material particles. [1895, p. 295]

Although this essay is a collaborative effort, the primary responsibility for the section on Hegel belongs to J. M. Woody and that on Heidegger to E. S. Casey.

Freud soon abandoned this neurophysiological program and declared forthrightly that, henceforth, "I shall remain upon psychological ground" (1900–01, p. 536). But similar reductionist motives remain prominent in his works, where the neuron's role as a naturalistic explanatory principle is supplanted by the conception of instinct or drive (*Trieb*) as a form of biological energy. The ambitions of the 1895 "Project" still echo in *An Outline of Psycho-Analysis,* posthumously published in 1938, where Freud declares that psychology is "a natural science like any other" (p. 158). In the light of such statements, it is easy to interpret Freudian psychoanalysis as a form of reductionist psychology that attempts to resolve everything human into a biological substrate of instinctual energies.

Jacques Lacan proposes an audacious alternative to this reductionist interpretation of Freud. He argues that what is central to Freud's view is not his official materialism, but a theory of symbolism. Lacan would thus substitute linguistics for biology as the scientific foundation and model for psychoanalysis, thereby ensuring that the human will be understood in terms of the human, since language is a uniquely human achievement. It is this proposal—that linguistics replace biology as the scientific paradigm for psychoanalysis—which links Lacan with the French structuralist school.

But if Lacan offers us an alternative to reductionistic versions of Freud and of psychoanalysis, it is not only because of his emphasis upon linguistics. It is also because his view is profoundly influenced by the philosophies of Heidegger and Hegel and, even more specifically, by Alexandre Kojève's provocative interpretation of Hegel's *Phenomenology of Spirit,* which had such a major impact upon French thinkers of Lacan's generation. Indeed, the influences of Heidegger and Hegel converge in Kojève, whose interpretation of Hegel's *Phenomenology* exhibits an original and exciting blend of Marxist and Heideggerian ingredients. Since many readers of Lacan are not familiar with Heidegger or Hegel, still less with Kojève's version of the *Phenomenology,* Lacan's Heideggerian allusions and frequent references to Hegel only aggravate the difficulty of wrestling with his hermetic prose style.

We will try to alleviate this difficulty by presenting some of the most salient ideas of Hegel and Heidegger that are important to understanding Lacan. Our purpose is not merely to clarify Lacan by tracing historical influences, however. We will also attempt to show how Lacan's assimilation of Hegel and Heidegger invites a reconsideration of the founding insights of Sigmund Freud in a less reductionistic way. Reductionism will give way to a dialectic that leads to a psychoanalysis no longer regarded, or regardable, as anything like a natural science.

Hegel

Lacan claims to be an orthodox Freudian, championing Freud's authentic meaning against the challenge of French phenomenology and the heretical ego psychology of the American Freudians. He attacks both the transparency of consciousness in Sartre's existential phenomenology and the primacy of the ego in American psychoanalytic theory, insisting that the ego is not the locus of truth and reality and autonomous control, but is rather a concretion of illusions, a source of "méconnaissances" or "misrecognitions" that must be dissolved in the course of psychoanalysis in order to liberate the authentic self, the "je" or "I."

Lacan finds Hegel a natural ally in these quarrels because Hegel, too, is a critic of consciousness and of the ego—not of ego psychology, of course, but of the ego-centered philosophies that have dominated modern European thought. These include Descartes's rational *cogito,* the introspective consciousness of English empiricism, and the autonomous, transcendental ego of Kant and Fichte. All are misconceptions insofar as they are founded in the idea of a purely epistemological ego—or "thinking being." For they thereby abstract not only from human activity and labor but also from the social, cultural, and historical conditions of human mentality. Thus, Kojève describes the program of *The Phenomenology of Spirit* somewhat dramatically by depicting it as Hegel's attempt to understand himself—*not* as a disembodied ego or Cartesian *cogito,* but as he sits at a table in Jena in 1806, writing the *Phenomenology* and hearing, in the distance, the cannon shots on the eve of the Battle of Jena, in which Napoleon defeated

Prussia. To understand himself, Hegel must understand what it is to philosophize at that historic moment, in a world in which Napoleon is about to end the Holy Roman Empire which Charlemagne had begun a thousand years before. But, Kojève asks,

> What is it to "understand" Napoleon? . . . Generally speaking, to understand Napoleon is to understand him in relation to the whole of anterior historical evolution, to understand the whole of universal history. Now, almost none of the philosophers contemporary with Hegel posed this problem for himself. And none of them, except Hegel, resolved it. For Hegel is the only one able to accept, and to justify, Napoleon's existence. . . . The others consider themselves obliged to *condemn* Napoleon, that is, to condemn the historical *reality;* and their philosophical systems—by that very fact—are all condemned by that reality. [*Introduction to the Reading of Hegel,* pp. 34–35; Kojève's italics]

These philosophers condemn Napoleon—and thereby themselves—because the abstract purity of the epistemological ego has been translated into a moralizing "beautiful soul" so obsessed with the purity of its own intentions that it does not *act*, but only passes judgment upon those who do—and of course Napoleon is the preeminent historic agent of the era. These philosophers are all words and no deeds, and by their very opposition to historical reality they show that their words are empty abstractions. They fail to understand Napoleon, as they fail to understand themselves, because they do not recognize that their abstract conception of themselves and Napoleon are both products of the culture of the Enlightenment, and that their condemnation of history is merely the verbal counterpart of what the Revolution and Napoleon are actively realizing by the destruction of the old order and the Holy Roman Empire. To understand Napoleon they would have to acknowledge this underlying identity of self and other, give up their abstract moralistic purity, and accept their own historicity.

Hegel insists that the individual who fails to recognize his own historicity and sets himself up as a pure, autonomous ego, independent of the customs and culture of his society and era, is a stranger to himself. Much of the work of *The Phenomenology of Spirit* is intended to dissolve such an illusory conception of the self as an abstract ego and bring the self-estranged consciousness to a full recognition of itself as both creature and creator of history. It is an enterprise that may well be compared with psychoanalysis and with Lacan's attack upon the ego as a source of mis-recognition and the alienation of the authentic subject. The easiest way to exhibit the Hegelian background of Lacan's view is to explore the parallel between these two programs for rescuing the self from its estrangement, or its "captivation by the ego," in Lacan's phrase.

The point of departure for Hegel's critique of ego philosophies is his analysis of consciousness, which culminates in a critique of the sort of naive scientific thinker who seeks to contemplate an objective world uncontaminated by subjectivity. This thinker still does not recognize that the mind plays an active role in knowledge, that the scientific object is a reflection of the scientific subject. The account ends with a strange passage on "die verkehrte Welt," an inverted, mirror world in which all scientific polarities are reversed—rather like speculations about a universe of antimatter in recent physics. Hegel carries this out to comic lengths to emphasize that the scientific consciousness must recognize itself in this mirror in order to get beyond mere consciousness and reach the level of self-consciousness. But self-consciousness emerges only if it is not nature that is the object of consciousness, but rather another self. Hegel therefore turns to the origins of consciousness in the relation to an alter ego:

> Self-consciousness is faced by another self-consciousness; it has come *out of itself.* This has a twofold significance: first, it has lost itself, for it finds itself as an *other* being; secondly, in doing so it has superseded the other, for it does not see the other as an essential being, but in the other sees its own self. [p. 111; Hegel's italics]

This image of the emergence of self-consciousness from the recognition of the self in a mirror, or in another self, is familiar to readers of Lacan. The point of departure for Lacan's critique of

ego psychology is his account of "the mirror stage"—the stage
when the infant, still uncoordinated and relatively powerless,
first achieves consciousness of itself by recognizing itself in an
object outside itself, its image in a mirror. According to Lacan,
this specular, mirror image of the self is "the matrix and first
outline of what is to become the ego,"[1] and since it shows the body
in reversed form, it presages the ego's role as a source of mis-
recognition and illusion.

What is not to be found in the looking glass, according to both
Hegel and Lacan, is any awareness of self as subjective agency.
The two agree that what the mirror does not reflect is the subject's
desire, which is the motive source of all human activity and is the
simplest, most primitive form of self-awareness. Kojève explains
that

> the man who attentively *contemplates* a thing, who wants to see
> it as it is without changing anything is "absorbed" so to speak
> by this contemplation—that is, by this thing. He forgets him-
> self. . . . [But] when he experiences a desire, when he is hun-
> gry, for example, and wants to eat . . . he necessarily be-
> comes aware of *himself*. Desire is always revealed as *my* desire.
> [p. 37; Kojève's italics]
>
> In contrast to the knowledge that keeps man in a passive
> quietude, Desire disquiets him and moves him to action.
> [p. 4]

Thus far, Lacan could concur on purely Freudian grounds—
and might defend his orthodoxy with references to Freud's discussions of Eros and Thanatos and the economics of the libido.
But what Lacan in fact does is to take over Hegel's analysis of
desire as interpreted and elaborated by Kojève. Hegel's analysis
focuses upon what distinguishes *human* desire from merely vital,
biological drives. If Lacan's version of Freudian theory and practice offers an alternative to reductionism, it is as much the result
of this adoption of Hegel's analysis of desire as it is of the linguis-

---

1. Laplanche and Pontalis (1973), pp. 250–52. For Lacan's own formulation, see
Écrits, pp. 1–7.

tic theory of the unconscious. Indeed, the linguistic and Hegelian themes may be regarded as necessary complements of one another. Paul Ricoeur objects to Lacan's interpretation of Freud because it "eliminates energy concepts in favor of linguistics" (p. 367, n. 37). By insisting upon a linguistic or semiotic theory of the unconscious, Ricoeur argues, Lacan and his followers are led to neglect the energetic, biological dimension of Freud's theory, the "economics" of the libido. But, Ricoeur insists, it is just this natural, energetic ingredient that is required to explain the difference between ordinary language and the symbolism of the unconscious. Ricoeur regards this as the critical juncture for the philosophical interpretation of Freud:

> For a philosophical critique, the essential point concerns what I call the place of that energy discourse. Its place, it seems to me, lies at the intersection of desire and language. . . . The intersection of the 'natural' and the 'signifying' is the point at which the instinctual drives are 'represented' by affects and ideas; consequently the coordination of the economic language and the intentional language is the main question of this epistemology and one that cannot be avoided by reducing either language to the other. [p. 395]

But, Ricoeur admits, the difficulty here centers in "the idea of an 'energy that is transformed into meaning.'" And he concedes that in order to resolve this difficulty, "it may be that the entire matter must be redone, perhaps with the help of energy schemata quite different from Freud's" (p. 395).

It is at just this point, "the intersection of the 'natural' and the 'signifying,'" that Lacan's adoption of Hegel's account of human desire plays such a decisive role. The linguistic interpretation of the unconscious seems to call for a complementary redefinition of desire in less naturalistic terms than those afforded by Freud's "energy discourse." Hegel's discussion of desire in *The Phenomenology of Spirit* supplies this complement by focusing upon how human desire transcends biological needs and organic drives. And if Ricoeur is correct in claiming that psychoanalysis is essentially a "hermeneutics of desire," then the adoption of the

Hegelian theory of desire is bound to have important implications for both the theory and the practice of the interpretation of the "language" of the unconscious. Kojève's elaboration of Hegel's analysis of desire might almost have been designed to address this enigma of how "energy is transformed into meaning" in a way that pertains directly to the problem of interpretation as it appears within the interpersonal setting of analysis.

In his commentary upon Hegel's discussion of desire, Kojève explains that the very being of man implies and presupposes a biological reality, an animal life and animal desire. But,

> if animal Desire is the necessary condition of Self-Consciousness, it is not the sufficient condition. [p. 4]

> The animal attains only Selbst-*gefühl*, *Sentiment* of self, but not Selbst-*bewusstsein*, Self-*Consciousness*—that is, it cannot *speak* of itself, it cannot *say* "I." . . . For Self-Consciousness to exist . . . there must be transcendence of self with respect to self as *given*. And this is possible, according to Hegel, only if desire is directed not toward a *given* being, but toward a *non*being . . . that is, toward another Desire, another greedy emptiness, another I. . . . Desire is human—or, more exactly, "humanizing," "anthropogenetic"—only provided that it is directed toward another *Desire* and an *other* Desire. [pp. 39–40; Kojève's italics]

> Thus, in the relationship between a man and a woman, for example, Desire is human only if the one desires, not the body, but the Desire of the other; if he wants "to possess" or "to assimilate" the Desire taken as Desire—that is to say, if he wants to be "desired" or "loved," or, rather, "recognized" in his human value, in his reality as a human individual. [p. 6]

Lacan takes up this analysis and elaborates it into a three-way distinction between *desire*; merely natural or biological *need*, which is mute; and *demand*, which is that peculiarly human demand for love that transcends all mere objects of satisfaction and transmutes them into proofs of love. Lacan reserves the word "desire" to refer to that transcendent, unconditional ingredient in the demand for love, the peculiarly human emptiness that cannot be satisfied by any object or proof of love. As Lacan puts it, "for both partners in the relation, both the subject and the Other, it is not enough to be subjects of need, or objects of love. . . . They must stand for the cause of desire" (*Écrits*, p. 287). So, Lacan explains, "if the desire of the mother *is* the phallus, the child wishes to *be* the phallus in order to satisfy that desire" (p. 289). And elsewhere he elaborates:

> The child, in his relation to the mother, a relation constituted in analysis not by his vital dependence on her, but by his dependence on her love, that is to say, by the desire for her desire, identifies himself with the imaginary object of this desire in so far as the mother herself symbolizes it in the phallus. [*Écrits*, p. 198]

Lacan's understanding of the significance of the phallus is crucial here. The phallus is not the physical organ, the penis or clitoris, but the symbolic object whose unveiling culminated the ancient mysteries. Lacan insists upon this special symbolic status: "The phallus is the privileged signifier of that mark in which the role of the logos is joined with the advent of desire (1977, p. 287). The phallus thus stands at that "intersection of desire and language" which Ricoeur describes as the philosophically critical crossroads of psychoanalytic theory. For Lacan, it marks the transcendence of human desire beyond organic need—a transcendence that is owing to language. It also stands for *jouissance,* that unconditional fulfillment or perfection of being which is the aim of a human desire that cannot be satisfied by any object because "the being of language is the non-being of objects" (p. 263). In effect, the phallus is the symbol of that movement whereby man surpasses the merely vital or biological toward a fulfillment that is forever wanted—and forever wanting—in human existence.

Hegel, too, had insisted that this distinctively human desire to be desired aims beyond every determinate need and seems even to defy any form of satisfaction. It is a desire to be desired as a desirer; *not* simply to satisfy a *need*, nor as an object of *love*, as Lacan says, but as a human subject who transcends every object or instinct or merely vital need. But an individual can only prove to the other that he *is* such a transcending subject by risking his life in conflict with another subject. Kojève explains:

> For man to be truly human, for him to be essentially and really different from an animal, his human Desire must actually win out over his animal Desire. . . . All the Desires of an animal are in the final analysis a function of its desire to preserve its life. Human Desire, therefore, must win out over this desire for preservation . . . [pp. 6–7.] In other words, Man will risk his biological *life* to satisfy his *nonbiological* desire. And Hegel says that the being that is incapable of putting its life in danger in order to attain ends that are not immediately vital—i.e., the being that cannot risk its life in a fight for *Recognition,* in a fight for pure *prestige*— is *not* a truly *human* being. [p. 41; his italics]

But one cannot extract recognition from a corpse! A struggle to the death can only end in impasse. If the struggle is to have any positive result, one of the two adversaries must surrender, abnegate his own desire in order to save his life and become a slave who labors to satisfy the desire of the other, the master. But the master cannot be fully satisfied by the recognition of a mere slave who has sacrificed his human autonomy to save his life. *Self*-consciousness is achieved only through consciousness of another self, an alter ego, and the master cannot encounter a fully human self in the slave. It is only the slave who encounters in the master, as his alter ego, a fully autonomous human being. But this otherness must be overcome; the self must recognize itself in its other. The master must acknowledge his dependence upon the slave, and the slave must recognize his own mastery. In fact, it is the slave who, by means of his labor, may eventually achieve satisfaction and recognition. The slave alters and reshapes the world through his work and thereby realizes and embodies his own subjective agency in the world. He can therefore *recognize* himself in that world. By laboring to satisfy the desire of the other, then, the slave *works through* his natural fear of death and realizes his freedom by mastering the natural world, thereby achieving self-recognition.

Lacan applies this analysis of the struggle for recognition and the master-slave relation to the development of the child and to the psychoanalytic process. The child desires to be desired—desires, symbolically, to *be* the phallus which the mother desires. But he must repress this desire under the prohibition of the paternal "No," or as Lacan puts it "in the Name of the Father," which signifies the socialization of the child, the acquisition of language, law, and culture whereby the individual becomes human. This subordination of desire to law and language is the locus of primal repression. The threat of castration is simply the apt symbol for this abnegation of the desire to be desired, symbolized by the desire to be the phallus. Lacan also finds here the source of the necessity which led Freud to "link the appearance of the signifier of the Father, as author of the Law, with death, even to the murder of the Father" (*Écrits*, p. 199).

Thus, according to Lacan, there is a "life and death struggle" at the origin of individual acculturation much like that which Hegel saw as the precondition of all human history. In both cases, this struggle leaves the desire for recognition unsatisfied, and the subsequent development—whether of the career of the individual or the history of the species—is plagued by tensions that betray the unresolved conflict whence it springs. Lacan writes:

> The concrete field of individual preservation . . . is structured in this dialectic of master and slave, in which we can recognize the symbolic emergence of the imaginary struggle to the death in which we earlier defined the essential structure of the ego. [*Écrits*, p. 142]

Lacan sees this same dialectic in psychoanalytic transference. He frequently characterizes the analytic relationship in just these Hegelian terms, describing it as a struggle for recognition or as a master-slave relation in which the analysand assumes the role of the slave, who agrees initially to undertake the "work" of analysis in order to satisfy the analyst-master. If the process is to be fruitful, however, the analyst must eventually eschew the role of master and help the analysand toward self-recognition through the labor of free association, thereby freeing an authentic "I" from captivation by the ego.

Of course, all of this must be taken metaphorically. In Lacan's case, nothing should be taken too literally—and Lacan himself remarks that Hegel's account describes "a mythical rather than a real genesis" (*Écrits,* p. 308). It is probably best to see Hegel's analysis of the struggle for recognition and the master-slave dialectic as his substitute for the Enlightenment's myth of the origin of human civilization in a social contract between autonomous, rationally self-interested egos. Kojève treats this dialectic as a metaphor for the whole of human history, in which the labor of the slave corresponds to the historical process of *Bildung,* or culture-building, wherein man both creates and alienates himself:

> The historical process, the historical becoming of the human being, is the product of the working Slave and not of the warlike Master. . . . Thanks to his work, *he* can become other; and thanks to his work, the *World* can become other. And this is what actually took place as universal history and, finally, the French Revolution and Napoleon show. [pp. 52–53]

And that brings us back to the beginning, to Hegel's effort to understand himself as he writes, hearing the sounds of Napoleon's cannon at Jena, and to his attempt to help the reader overcome his self-estrangement by appropriating his own historicity, recognizing himself as both creature and creator of history. It is, again, an undertaking which invites comparison with psychoanalysis, especially as Lacan describes it: "Analysis can have for its goal only the advent of a true speech and the realization by the subject of his history in his relation to a future" (*Écrits,* p. 88).

Yet for all the fertile parallels Lacan discovers between psychoanalysis and the program of Hegel's *Phenomenology,* the two enterprises are not the same, and he is well aware of how they differ. In Hegel's case, the task of reconciliation with his own historical reality requires an understanding of the whole of world history, or at least of how the history of the West has led to the confrontation between the German intellectual and the Napoleonic armies. Only the philosophical comprehension of the history that culminates in Napoleon will yield such self-understanding and reconciliation. Self-knowledge is not to be attained through the simple transparency of the Cartesian *cogito* or Kant's transcendental unity of apperception, for man is not an enduring substance, knowable through the contemplation of some timeless essential attributes. Man is a free agent and he cannot know *what* he is until he acts, since he constitutes himself through acting upon and altering his world. Man's essence is defined by his history, by what he has done, and that means that he can only come to know himself by alienating or othering himself, by building himself a world and then recognizing himself in that world of culture and history, understood as the product of his human deeds.

But the individual who fully recognizes all this, and understands that history is a human creation, is himself no longer a mere creature of history. *That* individual, of course, is Hegel himself. By fully understanding his own historicity, Hegel claims to transcend it, not by ascending to a realm of Platonic Ideas, nor by escaping into a timeless mystic unity, but precisely by insisting that man's freedom makes him radically temporal and historical; and yet to understand this history is to transcend it in a knowledge that is absolute because it grasps the truth of all the antecedent forms of consciousness and culture, and knows itself to be the product of those forms. It thereby comprehends the whole of history within itself. So, Hegel concludes,

> Spirit necessarily appears in Time, and it appears in Time just so long as it has not *grasped* its pure Notion, i.e., has not annulled Time . . . . Time, therefore, appears as the destiny and necessity of Spirit that is not yet complete within itself, the necessity to enrich the share which self-consciousness has in consciousness. [*Phenomenology*, p. 487]

Hegelian phenomenology and Lacanian psychoanalysis part company here. For Lacan would forswear such a claim to absolute knowledge, emphasizing that the analyst must abjure any comparable assertion of omniscience. And this is surely not because of any modesty on Lacan's part, but because of his conviction that there is no final insight or definitive version of truth to be had. If Lacan nevertheless acknowledges the radical historicity and temporality of human existence by insisting upon the roles of language, law, and culture in the constitution of the individual subject, he must avail himself of a different conception of human temporality, historicity, and culture than Hegel's. He found such an alternative conception ready to hand in the philosophy of Martin Heidegger.

Heidegger

For Lacan the human subject is something more than ego and even more than consciousness. At one point, Lacan is tempted to connect his view of the subject with Descartes's insofar as both seek certainty in the midst of doubt: "The subject," says Lacan, is always "looking for his certainty" (*Four Fundamental Concepts of Psycho-Analysis,* p. 129). He is a subject who is "supposed to know" (*le sujet supposé à savoir:* "posited as in the know") but who does *not* know because of the misunderstandings and mystifications in which he or she is embroiled in the imaginary register that begins with the infant's captivation by its reflection in the mirror. But it is just here that the parallel with Descartes collapses. For the Cartesian subject achieves certainty by recognizing its being through self-reflection, and can be defined with metaphysical precision as a *res cogitans,* an undivided thinking substance—whereas the subject of (and in) psychoanalysis has "wider bases" and is radically indeterminate: a subject always "split" and "fading" from itself in self-division (cf. *Four Concepts,* p. 126; *Écrits,* pp. 299, 313).

There are various sources of such splitting of the subject. They include the intrinsic incommensurabilities between the repressing and the repressed elements of the self, the signifier and the signified, language and speech, self and other, ego and Other. This split and divided condition of the subject, which Lacan signifies by the symbol $, means that the immediate reflective certainty of the Cartesian *cogito* is an illusion, a mis-recognition. And as this cleavage in the self is radical, it cannot be transcended or reconciled through the mediated self-recognition of Hegelian absolute knowledge.

Does this mean, as some have suspected, that the Lacanian

subject can be neither known nor defined? In fact, there are at least three ways to define this subject, all of which are explicitly philosophical and each of which contributes to an understanding of its radically divided character.

THE EFFECTS OF THE SIGNIFIER

The subject for Lacan is a speaking subject—or rather, a *spoken* subject, created by the play of the signifier. Instead of being a source of causal efficacy (as it is in nearly all substantialist/ personalist views), the subject is to be regarded as an effect—indeed, the primary effect—of speaking. And it is precisely at this juncture that the unconscious enters the scene:

> One should see in the unconscious the effects of speech on the subject—insofar as these effects are so radically primary that they are properly what determine the status of the subject as subject . . . . The unconscious is the sum of the effects of speech on a subject, at the level at which the subject constitutes himself out of the effects of the signifier. [*Four Concepts*, p. 126]

For all of the obvious origins of such a statement in Saussure, Jakobson, and Lévi-Strauss, each of whom offers evidence of the massive "effects of the signifier," it is also rooted in the philosophy of Heidegger, who has insisted on the primacy of language over the speaking subject in his extremely condensed formula, "language speaks" (*die Sprache spricht*). At best, human beings can serve only to guard and preserve the truth thus spoken. At worst, and more typically, they may abandon authentic meaning and subjectivity in a life dominated by the cliché and by everyday gossip. David Riesman once epitomized the heteronomy of such a life by describing it as "other-directed." Heidegger expresses the same theme by saying that this inauthentic, everyday subject is not *myself*, but the impersonal "one" (*das Man,* the equivalent of the French *on*).

Lacan articulates this theme by speaking of the dominance of the Other. In the last section of his 1957 essay "The Agency of the Letter in the Unconscious," entitled "The Letter, Being and the

Other," he speaks of "the radical heteronomy that Freud's discovery [of the unconscious] shows gaping within man" and of "this other to whom I am more attached than to myself" (*Écrits*, p. 172). This "Other," which Lacan distinguishes from any particular other by capitalization ("*le grand Autre*"), is not distinguishable from the signifying chain of speech in which it manifests itself in psychoanalysis; indeed, it is "the locus of the signifier" (p. 310). Hence Lacan's celebrated dictum, "The unconscious is the discourse of the Other" (p. 172). The unconscious is structured *as* a language because, and to the exact extent that, it is structured *by* language. Or, to put it another way: language provides the "structure and limit" (p. 56) of the field in which the subject comes-to-be, and this means above all the psychoanalytic subject.

THE ECSTATIC SELF

But what *is* this subject, after all, this being who is defined by language and who becomes Other to himself by being *in* language? "What constitutes me as subject is my question," remarks Lacan (*Écrits*, p. 86), echoing Heidegger's description of *Dasein* as a questioning being in the introduction to *Being and Time*. Questioning—whether of oneself, of other beings, or of Being itself— is itself a fundamental form of splitting within the subject, since it inexorably introduces a division between the questioner and the questioned, the known and the unknown. Lacan therefore speaks of the subject as "ex-centric," as alienated from himself. The philosophical origins of this conception of the subject again derive from Heidegger's analysis of subjectivity in *Being and Time*. In this work of 1927, Heidegger designates human existence as "Dasein": literally, being-there. To be-there is to ex-ist, to stand-out in one's being-in-the-world. Such ex-isting is a way in which *to-be:*

> The 'essence' of this entity [*Dasein*] lies in its 'to be' [*Zu-sein:* about to be, implying possibility]. . . . *The essence of Dasein lies in its existence.* . . . In each case Dasein *is* its possibility. [*Being and Time*, pp. 67–68; Heidegger's italics]

Dasein exists, then, by standing out—out from the world regarded as a collection of indifferent, present-at-hand particulars and out from itself as a centered substrate. As thus ex-centric and ex-static, Dasein stands out as being something other than its mundaneity or egocentricity would prescribe or predict; and it does so in two basic ways: (1) *Dasein* ex-ists by the *projection of existentially significant possibilities* through its understanding of the world and itself: an understanding that is essentially pro-jective by virtue of its fore-structure, through which it is ineluctably drawn into the hermeneutical circle of knowing projectively what it comes to know in detail in cognitive (and other forms) of inquiry; and (2) *Dasein* also stands out from itself by its *involvement with others* in the "with-world" of human sociality, especially in the crucial activity of "leaping ahead" in relation to others rather than "leaping in" for them by directly disburdening them of their anxiety or cares—where "leaping ahead" has remarkable affinities with psychoanalytic techniques of abstinence, silence, and empathic understanding. Such leaping ahead contrasts with the deadened and deadening passivity of *das Man* understood as the "they-self" which dictates conformity and submission.

TEMPORALITY

Basic to all these ex-centricities and making them possible is the temporality of the self. If the human subject could not distance itself from itself in time, it would live an unsplintered life of immediacy, of continuous bodily need and its gratification (whether actual or hallucinated). For the advent of demand and desire, there must be a power of projecting satisfactions in time— whether through memory or through anticipation of a wished-for object. Either way, whether I project toward a past or a future horizon, temporality exhibits itself in its radically differentiating role: as allowing me to differ from my present self, to be other than myself, to be self-alien in time.

Heidegger therefore defines temporality as "the primordial 'outside-of-itself' in and for itself" (*Being and Time*, p. 377). By this designation, he means to emphasize that the human experience of time cannot be confined to a succession of nows, arranged primly on some time-line. The series of now-points to which we are so often tempted to reduce temporal experience results from quantifying and shrinking a temporality that in and by itself is profoundly nonlinear. Such temporality, which belongs to *Dasein* precisely as ex-istent or standing outside its own self-enclosed ego, is termed "ecstatico-horizonal" by Heidegger. Each of the three main forms of temporality—past, present, and future—can be seen as an open horizon which we actively project out of our existential concerns and preoccupations. Each temporal horizon is *outside* the center or source of the projecting, whether as having-already-been, going-to-be, or making-present. As such, each is a possible mode of temporalization, of being-in-time ec-statically. But of the three modes, the future has priority: "The primary phenomenon of primordial and authentic temporality is the future" (p. 378). Why so? The reason is that in relation to the future, *Dasein* is outside itself, apart from itself, in the most radical way: its basic "to-be" character, as accomplished in the projection of possibilities, is realized most completely in relation to the future, which is indeterminately open and is the locus of one's being-toward-death. It is in and through such temporalization of its existence that *Dasein* is self-centrifugal: alienated from itself in the literal sense of being, in time, other than itself. This is not to be regretted, Heidegger thinks; indeed, it is the way in which we live out our human existence most authentically. Inauthenticity enters only when the diasporadic, spread-out and opened-up sense of temporality just described is closed down and confined to a mere sequence of nows—to sheer "within-time-ness" (*Innerzeitigkeit*), in contrast to the disjunctive, ecstatico-horizonal temporality of authentic *Dasein*.

What do such apparently arcane descriptions of human temporality have to do with psychoanalysis? Lacan finds that Heidegger's analysis applies directly to the practice of psychoanalysis because "time plays its role in analytic technique in several ways" (*Écrits*, p. 95). The most obvious temporal parameters of the analytic process are its duration as a whole and the length of each session.

Total duration. The length of analysis cannot be determined in advance. For the subject in treatment, the total time it will take "can only be anticipated . . . as indefinite" (*Écrits*, p. 95). Why is this? Lacan's immediate response is that the *temps pour comprendre*—the time required for understanding and bespeaking oneself as subjectivity—is strictly unpredictable. Lacan's phrase "anticipated as indefinite" evokes the very terms Heidegger used to describe the decisive notion of authentic temporality as involving being-toward-death (*Sein-zum-Tode*). Although death is the ending of life, Heidegger explains, it is neither a goal to be sought nor a terminal point to be merely awaited; it is the kind of thing we are always tending *toward,* yet may be either kept concealed from us or authentically anticipated (see *Being and Time,* p. 303). But since my death cannot be determined precisely in advance, in its exact character or position in the future, it is something I can only anticipate in an open-ended way, as "indefinite."

If the analytic experience is indeed analogous to being-toward-death, then it would be a grievous technical error to try to fix its end in advance. Freud attempted to do this in the case of the Wolf Man and came to regret it. Here the end was held out as definite, as something to be awaited and expected. This made the point of termination too determinate and produced what Lacan calls a "mirage," a "spatializing projection" (*Écrits,* pp. 95–96), because it destroyed the element of nonfixed standing-out which is an indispensable feature of Dasein's temporality. Since the subject of psychoanalysis is a genuinely temporal being, the analytic process must reflect this fact by becoming itself intrinsically indefinite in duration. It is in this sense, indeed, that psychoanalysis can be said to be "interminable," in Freud's term, which Lacan revealingly translates into French as "*indéfinie.*" To understand psychoanalysis as terminable in a definite, end-positing way is to transform its diffuse temporality into an alienated spatiality, and thus to foster "the vertigo of the domination of space" (p. 28).

Length of session. One of the most controversial features of Lacan's own practice has been his alteration of the length of the psychoanalytic session. The duration of this session is fixed by tradition at fifty minutes. Lacan finds the strict and unquestioning adherence to this time span suspiciously obsessional,[2] and has

2. Lacan himself seemed to regard his shortened sessions as frankly experimental and perhaps a thing of the past: "I would not have much to say about [such a matter] if I had not been convinced that, in experimenting with what have been called my short sessions, at a stage in my experience that is now concluded" (*Écrits,* p. 100). It is also to be noted that Lacan experimented with *lengthening* sessions.

advocated the seemingly arbitrary practice of terminating the session at the discretion of the analyst, reportedly after as little as several minutes.

We make no attempt to attack or defend this practice but wish only to point to its roots in Heidegger's contrast between human time and clock time. Although certainly useful for many purposes, clock time does not begin to reflect adequately the temporality of Dasein, much less of the unconscious. According to Heidegger, the time of clocks is the result of leveling down primordial temporality to a measurable (and measuring) public time that is impersonal and impartial. Lacan remarks that the advent of clock time "is relatively recent, since it goes back precisely to Huyghens' clock—in other words, to 1659—and the *malaise* of modern man does not exactly indicate that this precision is in itself a liberating factor for him" (*Écrits,* p. 98).

Lacan warns that strict observation of the fifty-minute rule may prove more oppressive than liberating. One is oppressed by the fateful inevitability with which one measured moment succeeds another until the set interval is marked off on some indifferent clock face. Indifference, indeed, is the heart of the matter:

> The indifference with which the cutting up of the 'timing' interrupts the moments of haste within the subject can be fatal to the conclusion towards which his discourse was being precipitated, or even fix a misunderstanding or misreading in it, if not furnish the pretext for a retaliatory ruse. [p. 99]

In order to make the inadequacy and oppressive indifference of the standard session tolerable, a patient may collude with clock time itself: submit to it, labor in it conscientiously, yet temporize all the while. This labor, observed most dramatically in obsessives, is "forced labor" whose motive lies in the awaited death of the analyst qua master (cf. *Écrits,* p. 26). But any such attitude toward death, whether it be one's own or another's, is manifestly inauthentic and deadens the analytic process itself through the patient's identification with the quasi-impendingly dead analyst. The patient lives "in the [expectation] of the master's death, from which moment he will begin to live, but in the meantime he identifies himself with the master as dead, and as a result of this he is himself already dead" (p. 100). This result, adds Lacan, is one of the aspects of the master-slave dialectic which Hegel did *not* describe but which is powerfully operative in psychoanalytic practice.[3]

The Vicissitudes of the Influences

Investigation of Lacan's Hegelian roots led us to turn to Heidegger; reflection upon his debt to Heidegger has now led us back to Hegel. But the ingression of these two influences in Lacan's thinking is not as conveniently complementary as this circle might suggest. A number of unresolved issues emerge from their convergence, and we shall pose these in order to set the stage for a discussion of how Lacan appropriates both influences in a psychoanalytic theory that is at once both deeply Freudian and strikingly original.

THE DISPLACEMENT OF CONSCIOUSNESS

The point at which the convergent influences of Hegel and Heidegger most obviously collide concerns the question of consciousness. There is no obvious way to harmonize their views on this subject, hence no way in which Lacan might integrate them in a higher synthesis. Although Hegel certainly does not conceive of consciousness as the consciousness of the Cartesian ego, he is nevertheless ineradicably committed to the concept of consciousness, or more exactly and significantly, to a dialectic which transforms all consciousness into *self*-consciousness. *The Phenomenology of Spirit* traces an evolution of forms of consciousness in which whatever consciousness takes to be an independent substance is shown to be only an object-for-consciousness and thereby appropriated by self-consciousness. Hegel even says that mind or spirit

3. "The slave has given way in face of the risk of death in which mastery was being offered to him in a struggle of pure prestige. But since he knows that he is mortal, he also knows that the master can die. From this moment on he is able to accept his labouring for the master and his renunciation of pleasure in the meantime; and, in the uncertainty of the moment when the master will die, he waits" (*Écrits*, p. 99).

is precisely this process of transforming "Substance into Subject, the object of *consciousness* into the object of *self-consciousness*. . . . The movement is the circle that returns into itself, the circle that presupposes its beginning and reaches it only at the end" (p. 488; Hegel's italics).

Heidegger, by contrast, deliberately rejects the language of consciousness in *Being and Time* because he believes that the entire "epoch" of post-Cartesian philosophy, including Hegel and Husserl, has been too self-centered on the metaphysics of the subject. Much as Lacan claims that psychoanalysis must move away from the narcissistic discourse of the empty word—from "the mirage of the monologue" (*Écrits*, p. 41), which is nevertheless its natural and necessary beginning point—so Heidegger demands that pure consciousness, the very foundation of the Cartesian *cogito* and of Husserl's phenomenological reduction, be transcended in the existential analytic of *Dasein,* whose structures of "being-in" (state-of-mind, understanding, discourse, and fallenness) do not include the least vestige of pure consciousness.

It is not surprising that Lacan should side with Heidegger in this dispute. Just as Freud had excoriated philosophers generally for conflating mind with consciousness, so Lacan takes Hegel to task for not allowing more adequately for the dispossession of consciousness, its displacement or "subversion" by the subject of desire:

> Freud's discovery was to demonstrate that this verifying process [i.e., that the real is rational] authentically attains the subject only by decentering him from the consciousness-of-self, in the axis of which the Hegelian reconstruction of the phenomenology of mind maintained it. [*Écrits*, p. 80]

For Hegel, Lacan argues, "the subject knows what he wants" (p. 301) from the very outset. Since whatever is recognized by self-consciousness was already present to consciousness, the end is present from the beginning, and perfect self-consciousness is therefore "the fundamental hypothesis of this whole process. [It] is named, in effect, as being the substratum of this process: [it] is called the '*Selbstbewusstsein*', the being conscious of self, the fully conscious self" (p. 296). But for Lacan the subject cannot know what he wants at the outset: his very existence consists in a systematic *méconnaisance*. The very process of psychoanalysis is one of coming to know one's desiring self from a state of initial symptomatic ignorance; it is a matter of the recognition of repressed desire, a recognition which requires the mediating role of the analyst as the foil from which the expression of one's own self-unknown desire returns in a reversed form that lays it bare (*Écrits*, p. 85). Another way of putting this is to stress the essential opacity of the "I" in contrast with the putative clarity of consciousness:

> The promotion of consciousness as being essential to the subject in the historical after-effects of the Cartesian *cogito* is for me the deceptive accentuation of the transparency of the 'I' in action at the expense of the opacity of the signifier that determines the 'I'; and the sliding movement [*glissement*] by which the *Bewusstsein* serves to cover up the confusion of the *Selbst* eventually reveals, with all Hegel's own rigour, the reason for his error in *The Phenomenology of Spirit*. [p. 307]

Hegel too naively assumed that the self finds complete and transparent expression in the language and culture it produces and can attain full satisfaction and freedom by recognizing itself therein. But Freud discovered that the conscious significance may only dissimulate the subject's real desire in order to satisfy the demands of a superego imposed upon the subject by the very acquisition of language and culture.

Here we cannot speak seriously of any strict complementarity between Hegel and Heidegger, for it is not a question of what would fill out consciousness to make some larger whole, but of that which undermines the self-confidence and self-certainty of consciousness itself. For Heidegger and Lacan, consciousness is self-extirpating, not self-exfoliating.

TOTALITY

The mention of "whole" brings us to another major confrontation between Lacan's primary philosophical progenitors. For Hegel, the truth lies in the whole—in the totality of the philosophical system which is attained in absolute knowledge. The truth of any given stage of development always lies in the necessarily more ample successor stage, and ultimately in the totality of stages. Heidegger recognizes no such cumulative dialectic; *Being and Time* presents us with a scattered set of *Dasein*'s existential structures. This results in such a disconcerting array of features that Heidegger is driven to draw them together under such englobing rubrics as "care" and temporality. But neither care nor temporality represents a higher level, or a more truthful phase, of fundamental ontology: in the text they function mainly as modes of encirclement and repetition. No progressive or even strictly successive movement is realized in the pages of *Being and Time*, much less in Heidegger's later writings.

Once again, Heidegger and Lacan are natural colleagues compared with Hegel; but this time Lacan goes still further in his dissociation from the latter. What is most primordial and most valued is not systematic totality but dispersal or discontinuity itself—in a word, *difference* rather than *identity*. Lacan's phrases for such ur-difference include references to the subject's "original splitting," to his "radical heteronomy," to his status as a "discontinuity in the real" (*Écrits*, pp. 28, 172, 299). The critical factor in the determination of the subject in psychoanalysis always occurs in the form of a disconnection or "cut" (*coupure*) in the conscious chain of signifiers:

> Discontinuity, then, is the essential form in which the unconscious first appears to us as a phenomenon—discontinuity, in which something is manifested as a vacillation. Now, if this discontinuity has this absolute, inaugural character in the development of Freud's discovery, must we place it—as was later the tendency with analysts—against the background of a totality?
>
> Is the *one* anterior to discontinuity? I do not think so, and everything I have taught in recent years has tended to exclude this need for a closed *one*. . . . You will grant me that the *one* that is introduced by the experience of the unconscious is the *one* of split, of the stroke, of rupture. [*Four Concepts*, pp. 25–26]

The bar of repression is a strictly unsurpassable barricade which splits the subject (\$) just as the bar (_____) splits the sign into signifier and signified ($\frac{S}{s}$).

What is the subject thus split *into*? Not into id, ego, and super-ego, as on Freud's structural model. Instead, the split finds its paradigm in Heidegger's distinction between the "ontic" and the "ontological," between particular beings and Being. Heidegger claims that our preoccupation with particular beings covers up and conceals the question of the meaning of Being. Similarly, Lacan distinguishes between the Other and others. The Other is the unconscious regarded as "the pure subject of the signifier" (*Écrits*, p. 305), whereas others are the counterparts of the ego: any object, including other persons qua objects, with which the subject may affiliate in a real, imaginary, or symbolic mode. The difference between Other and other is constituted by the bar of repression, much as attention to particular beings veils the meaning of Being, according to Heidegger. In Heidegger's later writings, "difference" and "rift" emerge as still more central than in *Being and Time*, and these concepts have influenced not only Lacan, but Merleau-Ponty, Deleuze, and Derrida. Common to all these thinkers is an emphasis on differentiation at the expense of totalization, which distinguishes them sharply from Hegel, whose entire system is epitomized in the idea that "the truth is the whole."

DEATH

Yet Heidegger himself recognized quite clearly that his emphasis upon the existential and ec-static raises serious problems about *Dasein*'s totalization. The second division of *Being and Time*, the analysis of temporality, begins with a section entitled "The Seeming Impossibility of Getting Dasein's Being-a-Whole into our Grasp Ontologically and Determining its Character." Here we read that "as long as *Dasein is* as an entity, it has never reached its 'wholeness.' But if it gains such 'wholeness,' this gain becomes the utter loss of Being-in-the World" (p. 280). It is in answer to this paradox, indeed, that Heidegger embarks upon his analysis of being-toward-death as the only way in which *Dasein*'s being-a-whole is realizable. Nevertheless, one cannot *achieve* totality in

death, since by dying one ceases to exist. Being-a-whole is therefore "realizable" only as something continually receding, not as
an end-state or as a completion "still outstanding" which we could
expect or await. Still, being-toward-death is the most complete
and most authentic way in which one can be ahead-of-oneself.
But what one is ahead *for* or *about* is not the event of dying—which
is mere "perishing"—but something which is inherently indefinite, as we have seen. It is a matter of the "possible impossibility"
of one's existence, and one is almost perversely advised to be
resolute about that which, by its very nature, can never be definitively resolved. If Hegel allows spirit to achieve its end in absolute
knowledge, *Dasein* is consigned to being toward an end which it
cannot attain without ceasing to ex-ist and losing its "to-be" character. Being-toward-death is thus a strangely nonfinal form of
finalism, a nontelic teleology.

Contrast with this suspended state the situation at the end of
The Phenomenology of Spirit. In this finale, finalism is genuinely
finalistic. There is nothing more to be anticipated, since the end is
all encompassing. Each prior stage of the dialectic of self-consciousness has been taken up into the next in such a way that
nothing has been wholly lost. Hence spirit can be said to survive
the demise of each of its preceding avatars and to reach a decisive
culmination in absolute knowledge.

This epitomizes Hegel's own account of the acceptance of
death. Whereas natural life reaches its limit and end in death,
human existence transcends nature in taking the negativity of
death into itself and transmuting it into "the labor of the negative." In human culture and history, the fact and fear of death are
subordinated to the cumulative development of mind or spirit,
which is self-limiting and self-transcending. Death is "of all things
the most dreadful," Hegel writes:

> But the life of spirit is not the life that shrinks from death and
> keeps itself untouched by devastation, but rather the life that
> endures it and maintains itself in it. It wins its truth only
> when, in utter dismemberment, it finds itself. . . . . Spirit is
> this power only by looking the negative in the face and tarry-
> ing with it. This tarrying with the negative is the magic power

that converts it into being. This power is identical with what we earlier called the subject. [p. 19]

Thus, although Hegel argues that "it is only through staking one's life that freedom is won" (p. 114), freedom cannot be realized if one's life is actually lost, but only through the ongoing labors of the slave and his or her several historical permutations. Spirit "finds its truth" when it re-collects itself from this utter dismemberment in an absolute knowledge which is the appropriation of its own history and in which time itself is overcome and annulled. Such a result would be unthinkable in *Being and Time,* whose last sentence makes time the unsurpassable "horizon of Being" (p. 488).

The most important disparity between Hegel's and Heidegger's views on death, however, emerges from attempting to answer the question, *Whose* death is at stake here? For Heidegger, death is "my ownmost possibility" (p. 303). Since no one else can accomplish it for me, this possibility is preeminently my own and consequently "nonrelational" (p. 303). The authentic anticipation of death therefore "individualizes *Dasein* down to itself" (p. 308), summoning me out of everyday preoccupations and the anonymity of *das Man.* Being-toward-death is therefore the ultimate expression of the "mineness" (*Jemeinigkeit*) which is as primordial a characteristic of *Dasein* as existence itself (cf. p. 67). In psychoanalytic nomenclature, it is a matter of something strictly intrapsychic, of something one must come to know in one's essential aloneness.

For Hegel, by contrast, the acceptance of death is achieved through relation to another self—in the struggle for recognition—and the possibility of death becomes entangled in the interpersonal dialectic of the master-slave relation. Wherever the theme of death recurs in *The Phenomenology of Spirit,* it proves an occasion for a movement beyond the solitude of the mortal person toward community, toward recognizing that the truth of spirit is not "I," but "We."[4] In regard to this fundamental issue, Lacan

4. "Spirit is . . . this absolute substance which is the unity of the different independent self-consciousnesses which in their opposition enjoy perfect freedom and independence; 'I' that is 'We' and 'We' that is 'I' " (*The Phenomenology of Spirit,* p. 110).

sides with Hegel. The psychoanalytic situation is a scene of interlocution and is thus radically interpersonal and never reducible to two separate selves encountering each other. The we-ness of transference, for example, is confirmed by the fact of countertransference and by the dialectic engendered by the two transferential events. In contrast with the authentic individual's resolute but lonely anticipation of death, Lacan urges that the dialectic whereby the subject "brings his solitude to realization, be it in the vital ambiguity of immediate desire or in the full assumption of his being-for-death," is "not individual" (*Écrits*, p. 105). However solitary the individual's mortal end, the end of psychoanalysis is a "We," not an "I": "The question of the termination of analysis is that of the moment when the satisfaction of the subject finds a way to realize itself in the satisfaction of everyone—that is to say, of all those whom this satisfaction associates with itself in a human undertaking" (p. 105).

But if Lacan here agrees with Hegel that the goal is a personal truth or satisfaction that is at the same time intersubjective, he is not thereby tempted to endorse Hegel's claim that the truth lies in the whole and is to be achieved in an absolute knowledge which comprehends all particular truths within itself. Psychoanalysis can promise no such consummate truth. The Hegelian insistence upon the intersubjective must be tempered by the Heideggerian denial of totality. In the absence of the absolute knowledge of Hegel's self-knowing and self-known spirit, there is only the unending, indefinite search for a certainty which will never be attained as such. This is why psychoanalysis must find a third way between, or beyond, Hegel and Heidegger:

> Of all the undertakings that have been proposed in this century, that of the psychoanalyst is perhaps the loftiest, because the undertaking of the psychoanalyst acts in our time as a mediator between the man of care and the subject of absolute knowledge. [*Écrits*, p. 105]

$$\frac{LACAN}{freud}$$

In what way does psychoanalysis deserve this lofty office? What is lacking in these two great philosophical visions of truth, of self-discovery, and of reconciliation that can only be achieved through psychoanalysis? In the end Lacan dismisses both Hegelian and Heideggerian resolutions as impossible or inadequate. Why?

The answer lies in Freud's "Copernican step" (*Écrits,* p. 295), in the discovery of a dimension of the mind which transforms the human condition into a riddle: the unconscious. This is what is missing from both philosophical resolutions, and what foredooms any strictly philosophical quest for self-knowledge. Only psychoanalysis can make up for this lack, because only psychoanalysis offers a hermeneutics of the unconscious.

But the unconscious is not merely a cryptogram to be deciphered, whose interpretation would yield that absolute knowledge which Hegel promoted or the overcoming of alienation which Heidegger portrayed as the task of authentic existence. The unconscious is not simply an unknown realm to be incorporated into a more complete version of absolute knowledge, nor a level of man's being to be uncovered by a more fundamental ontology. The problem reaches much deeper. The existence of the unconscious means that the splitting of the subject, which begins with the infant's discovery of his image in the mirror, is as insurmountable for Lacan as it is for Sartre. The unity of the self in philosophical self-reflection is only a permutation of the reflected unity that stems from the situation wherein the infant, still subjectively disjointed, espies in the mirror a specular self having an imaginary unity, but wherein the subject of desire does not appear. This is because a desire is a *lack,* a want-to-be which cannot appear in an image; it can only refer to what is missing, to the object wanted, or, in this instance, to the very unity and coordination which are still lacking in the infant (see *Écrits,* p. 315). Nor do the mere maturation of the cortex and the development of motor skills guarantee integral *psychic* wholeness through natural organic development. The discrepancy between a disparate, incomplete subject and its imaged unity only anticipates a more profound splitting of the subject due to "the agency of the letter," to the subject's entrance into the symbolic order. This subjection of the subject to the effects of the signifier only replaces the image of the body in the mirror with the "I," a shifty word whose unity is all the more deceptive in that it is only a "shifter" which does not signify the self at all, but only designates whoever is speaking (*Écrits*, p. 298), and is therefore as indifferent to individuality as Heidegger's anonymous "one." Pursued further, this symbolic path will lead to the ego ideal, which does not represent the true subject, but only captivates him once more.

But to say that what is not present in these imaginary or symbolic representations is the self-as-desiring does not mean that what is lacking is the economics of the libido understood as the biological energetics of organic instinct. All this has only to do with *need*, which is prehuman. The effects of the signifier "proceed from a deviation of man's needs from the fact that he speaks, in the sense that insofar as his needs are subjected to demand, they return to him alienated" (*Écrits*, p. 286). The task of psychoanalysis is not to discover Rousseau's natural man beneath the brittle shell of a culture which imprisons him. Even if that were possible, analysis would not thereby liberate anything like a "noble savage," but the savagely patricidal brothers of Freud's *Totem and Taboo*. In any case, such a retrogression is not possible, because the natural man, uninfected by culture, is not a man at all, is not yet human, according to Lacan. And when it comes to man, purely organic need or natural instinct is as much a myth in Freud's eyes as was the natural man by Rousseau's own admission. "Instincts," says Freud, "are mythical entities, magnificent in their indefiniteness" (1933, p. 95). Moreover, as Hegel argued, the natural man's desire is not human desire because it is solipsistic, aimed only at consuming the object or using the other for his own solitary gratification (albeit a certain cunning of nature may in turn use his private pleasure to perpetuate the species).

But haven't we now returned to the beginning of this entire discussion, where we argued that Lacan simply adopts Hegel's analysis of desire instead of Freud's "energy discourse"? We have indeed insofar as Lacan persistently asserts that man's desire is the desire to be desired, thereby adhering to Hegel's analysis of desire. In fact, it is not Lacan but *Hegel* who departs from this very analysis. He does so not by abandoning his own view, but by sublating or transcending desire itself. For Hegel, desire is only the most immediate form of self-consciousness. Whether as hunger, thirst, or lust, it is self-feeling, a form of self-awareness we share with other animals. It becomes truly human only as the desire to be desired, when need becomes subjected to demand. But in either case it is only the most primitive form of self-consciousness, and is transcended through labor and history. Desire is not therein abandoned, but *aufgehoben,* surpassed and preserved. Thus desire is sublimated, taken up into history, which Hegel insists is only motivated by passion and self-interest (albeit a certain cunning of reason may transform private ambition into a means of realizing human truth). Following Kojève's metaphor, we could say that all of history is a permutation of the labor of the slave, who subordinates his own desire to that of the master, sacrificing human desire and pleasure to the fear of death, but finally finding satisfaction by recognizing himself in the objects produced by his labor—just as Hegel claimed to find absolute knowledge by recognizing world history as the progressive realization of that same absolute knowledge.

But for Lacan this is all *méconnaisance,* like identifying with one's own image in the mirror, since the subject can never be found adequately reflected in any object. There is no redemption or reconciliation to be had through history because the subject of desire can never be absorbed or *aufgehoben* in history, but only subverted or repressed there. In Lacanian language, Hegel attempted to absorb desire into demand, which is established by the *Logos,* in the realm of language, wholly mediated by symbolism and governed by the law of the signifier. Lacan agrees with Ricoeur to the extent that he holds that desire can never be entirely translated into demand, or strictly identified with the linguistic order. But at the same time, as we have just seen, he insists that desire can never be reduced to the merely natural, to biological need. Hence, in response to criticism of the Hegelian themes in his work, Lacan asserts that "far from ceding to a logicizing reduction where it is a question of desire, I find its irreducibility to demand the very source of that which also prevents it from being reduced to need" (*Écrits,* p. 302). What can this mean?

It means that the unconscious is not the hiding place of the natural man, and, further, is not to be confused with the cultural unconscious, wherein are stored such historical treasures as our unexamined beliefs, our tacit values, and the laws of our native language. It is no more a subterranean reservoir of volcanic emotional energy than it is the cerebral storehouse of the rules of a Chomskian transformational grammar. Lacan defines desire straightforwardly as that which rises out of the discrepancy between need and demand: "Thus desire is neither the appetite for satisfaction, nor the demand for love, but the difference which arises from the subtraction of the first from the second, the phenomenon of their splitting (*Spaltung*)" (*Écrits*, p. 287).

It is just here that we reach the origin of the dialectic of desire. Desire belongs *neither* to the natural *nor* to the symbolic order. It is situated at the intersection of the natural and the signifying, but neither the natural nor the signifying is left uninfected by the encounter. Desire arises at this intersection like a *herm,* that phallic post which the ancient Greeks erected at crossroads and dedicated to Hermes, the messenger of the gods and hence the patron of hermeneutics, the art or science of interpreting symbolism. We have already noted Lacan's insistence that the phallus is not an organ but a signifier, and this Hermetic function reminds us that the mysteries marked at this crossroads are not simply those of the barnyard or the birds and the bees, that the messenger of the gods is also present there. For the phallus points toward a *jouissance,* a fullness of being that is not to be attained through purely organic pleasures alone. Such pleasures, Lacan affirms, are transient satisfactions that may fulfill a need or answer the demand for proofs of love; but desire moves beyond the pleasure principle:

> Pleasure limits the scope of human possibility—the pleasure principle is a principle of homeostasis. Desire, on the other hand, finds its boundary, its strict relation, its limit, and it is in the relation to this limit that it is sustained as such, crossing the threshold imposed by the pleasure principle. [*Four Concepts,* p. 31]

This "strict relation" of desire to its limit refers to the internal bond between desire and the Law, which refers in the first instance to the injunction against incest operative in the oedipal situation. But Lacan finds in this very situation a set of relations which go beyond the specific prohibition against incest, something "indestructible" (*Four Concepts*, p. 31) escaping both temporality and historicity. These relations comprise a *structure* (see *Écrits*, p. 105) which transcends "culturalism"—and thus undercuts the dialectic of spirit—just because it represents the encounter between a needful organism and culture. For any culture inevitably imposes its own unnatural order, that of the signifier, upon the bodily subject. The incest taboo is only the nexus at which these two dimensions of human existence, the natural and the signifying, most conspicuously intersect.

Lévi-Strauss has assiduously demonstrated the same dialectic of nature and culture everywhere—at the intersection of the raw and the cooked, in the origin of table manners, and so forth. But Lacan scarcely needed the help of other French structuralists to discover this generalization of the oedipal conflict, since Freud had already made it the topic of an arresting analysis in *Civilization and its Discontents*. Lacan urges that the father in the oedipal triangle is not the actual father, but must be understood as a signifier, as "the Name of the Father." As such, he is not the one who provides for biological needs nor the one who might respond to the demand for love. It is the *dead* Father who "constitutes the law of the signifier" (*Écrits*, p. 217; cf. also pp. 199, 310). It is here that death insinuates itself into the Lacanian concept of desire in a veritable *Liebestod*. No longer a matter of an imminent being-toward-death to be authentically anticipated nor of an absolute master to be overcome by history, death enters as a condition of language:

> So when we wish to attain in the subject what was before the serial articulations of speech, and what is primordial to the birth of symbols, we find it in death, from which his existence takes on all the meaning it has. It is in effect as a

> desire for death that he affirms himself for others . . . and
> no being is ever evoked by him except among the shadows of
> death. [*Écrits*, p. 105]

The birth of symbols spells the death of things, since to begin to deal with the world symbolically is to enter into a world of meanings which mediate all human consciousness. The thing is thereby relegated to the status of that-which-is signified, as all direct awareness of things falls under the shadow of the signifier. Initiation into the Hermetic mysteries of the word therefore means "dying to the world" in a truly Socratic manner: "Thus the symbol manifests itself first of all as the murder of the thing, and this death constitutes in the subject the eternalization of his desire" (p. 104).

The subject's desire is both eternalized and subverted by the Father's signifying strictures, his prohibiting Law—the law of the signifier—with the result that the desiring subject is constituted as a subverted subject. Lacan calls such superimposing of the cultural upon the natural "primal repression" (in Freud's term) and holds it to be the very origin of the unconscious. But Lacan adds that it is also the origin of desire:

> That which is alienated in needs constitutes an *Urverdrän-
> gung* (primal repression), an inability, it is supposed, to be
> articulated in demand, but it reappears in something it gives
> rise to that presents itself in man as desire (*das Begehren*).
> [*Écrits*, p. 286]

Hence the law of the signifier sets up a bar dividing the subject, and is both constitutive and subversive of desire. It also bars the way to *jouissance,* that primordial union with the Mother whose recovery is prohibited by the paternal "No" and which signifies that completion of being which is forever inaccessible to the split subject. In this way, the relation of desire to its limit, upon which Lacan places so much emphasis, expresses an inescapable antinomy that is the final source of the dialectic of desire:

> But we must insist that *jouissance* is forbidden to him who
> speaks as such, although it can only be said between the lines

for whoever is subject of the Law, since the Law is grounded
in this very prohibition [*Écrits*, p. 319]

It is for this reason that the phallus, the *herm* erected at the
intersection of the natural and the signifying, comes to be conceived as the supreme signifier, the signifier of signifiers: "the
privileged signifier of that mark in which the role of the logos is
joined with the advent of desire" (*Écrits*, p. 287). For the phallus is

> itself a sign of the latency with which any signifiable is struck,
> when it is raised (*aufgehoben*) to the function of signifier. The
> phallus is the signifier of this *Aufhebung* itself, which it inau-
> gurates (initiates) by its very disappearance. That is why the
> demon of *Aidos* (*Scham*, shame) arises at the very moment
> when, in the ancient mysteries, the phallus is unveiled. [p.
> 288]

Or rather we should say that the phallus is the signifier of the bar
that separates the signifier from the signified in Saussure's for-
mula for signification $\frac{s}{s}$ ($\frac{\text{signifier}}{\text{signified}}$), which Lacan recasts as $\frac{S}{s}$ to
emphasize the dominance of the signifier. There is no trespassing
of this *barre*, which is ultimately that of *Urverdrängung*. The way is
barred, even if the bar can be said to withdraw once it is revealed.
The phallus signifies this bar in its simultaneously repressing and
revealing role: "it then becomes the bar which, at the hands of this
demon, strikes the signified, marking it as the bastard offspring
of this signifying concatenation" (p. 288). Herein lies the origin of
the split subject, barred from the urgent finalism of the desiring
self.

To invoke the phallus is also, and necessarily, to raise the question of castration. Castration, or more exactly its threat, is the
final undercutting of finality. It arises, first of all, in the under-
mining of oedipal triumph; but it remains potently present in the
sequel to this first splitting of the subject from his or her own
desire. For this sequel involves the establishment *from within* of
the very same limit, Law, or Name of the Father which is the
dyadic Other of desire. All of these belong under the heading of
the phallus and together give "the ratio of desire" (*Écrits*, p. 288).
But it is castration which *enforces* this ratio by barring *jouissance*:

> What analytic experience shows is that, in any case, it is castration that governs desire, whether in the normal or the abnormal. . . .
>
> Castration means that *jouissance* must be refused, so that it can be reached on the inverted ladder of the Law of desire. [*Écrits*, pp. 323–24]

The dialectic of desire shows it to be the desire of the Other: which means that it is marked indelibly by the play of the signifier, the intervention of language. This signifying play is dialectical to start with by virtue of its intersubjective source in the oedipal conflict; it becomes a matter of internal dialectic when the dissolution of this conflict leads to the installation of the Law within. But, as we have seen earlier, it can become interpersonal again in and through the process of analysis, when the desire of my Other rejoins the desire of other Others as mediated by the analyst, who is Other to myself. In the end, then, the dialectic of desire is intersubjective, and Hegel is supported against Heidegger. Heidegger is in turn borne out, however, in his conception of the subject as subordinate to language, as a bespoken subject who is in the end more the creature than the creator of language. What Lacan hastens to add, though, is that being bespoken is being broken—broken apart by the signifiers whose proper locus is to be found in the Other. The "eclipse of the subject" is in fact "closely bound up with the *Spaltung* or splitting that [the subject] suffers from its subordination to the signifier" (*Écrits*, p. 313).

But this splitting of the speaking subject is itself a reflection of "the division immanent in desire" (p. 289), a division which takes us back finally to Freud, the repressed influence in this essay. For it is Freud who proposed the leading hypotheses of primal repression and the castration complex, both of which are ultimately responsible for desire's diremption and hence for the splitting of the subject understood psychoanalytically. If the bar between "S" and "s" is raised in partial revelation by the Hermetic phallus, it is reimposed in a decidedly downward direction by that *Urverdrängung* and threat of castration which keep death at the doorstep of desire, Thanatos at the threshold of Eros. And the subject? His being is split irremediably between demand and need, with desire as the quotient of their difference.

Freud, the long-since-dead father of psychoanalysis, had already reached the reluctant conclusion that civilization and discontent are inseparable, that the subjection of man to culture foredooms him to what Hegel called "the unhappy consciousness," the "consciousness of self as a dual-natured, merely contradictory being" (p. 126). Lacan reinforces Freud's grim conclusion that the contradiction is insuperable, that history can promise no final reconciliation, no splendid synthesis, not even an arena for the attainment of authenticity: cuttings and splittings, human lives in tatters, are all that remain in this darkened vision.

But Lacan's own contribution is not to be subverted by the vicissitudes of his powerful influences. His claim to be the only orthodox interpreter of Freud in an age of heresy ironically disguises the originality which his conception of the dialectic of desire introduces into psychoanalytic theory. Nevertheless, his position is profoundly Freudian, and any assessment of Lacan's significance must acknowledge the Name of the Father of psychoanalysis as the repressed signifier which returns as only the repressed can return: inscribed symbolically and symptomatically, written over and overwritten, in that uniquely vexing set of signifiers whose name is *Écrits*.

REFERENCES

Freud, S. *Standard Edition of the Complete Psychological Works*. London: Hogarth, 1953–74.
    "Project for a Scientific Psychology" (1895), vol. 1.
    The Interpretation of Dreams (1900–01), vols. 4–5.
    New Introductory Lectures on Psycho-Analysis (1933), vol. 22.
    An Outline of Psycho-Analysis (1938), vol. 23.
Hegel, G. W. F. *The Phenomenology of Spirit* (1807). Translated by A. V. Miller. Oxford: Oxford University Press, 1977.
Heidegger, M. *Being and Time* (1927). Translated by J. Macquarrie and E. Robinson. New York: Harper, 1962.

———. *Vorträge und Aufsätze.* Pfullingen: Neske, 1954.

Kojève, A. *Introduction to the Reading of Hegel: Lectures on "The Phenomenology of Spirit"* (1933–39). Edited by A. Bloom. Ithaca: Cornell University Press, 1980.

Lacan, J. *Écrits: A Selection* (1966). Translated by A. Sheridan. New York: Norton, 1977.

———. *The Four Fundamental Concepts of Psycho-Analysis* (1973). Translated by A. Sheridan. New York, Norton, 1978.

Laplanche, J., and Pontalis, J.-B. *The Language of Psychoanalysis.* Translated by D. Nicholson-Smith. New York: Norton, 1973.

Ricoeur, P. *Freud and Philosophy: An Essay on Interpretation* (1965). Translated by D. Savage. New Haven: Yale University Press, 1970.

6

Hegel as Lacan's Source for Necessity in Psychoanalytic Theory

WILFRIED VER EECKE

The project of Lacan has been described in different ways. Lacan is said to have returned to the *real* Freud. He is said to have used modern sciences of man (linguistics, structural anthropology) in order to provide a theoretical basis for psychoanalytic insights. He is also said to have given psychoanalysis a more rigorous scientific status.

Of these three descriptions of the Lacanian oeuvre, it is the third one which will hold our attention here. Giving scientific status to a discipline means among other things to assign some sort of *necessity* to phenomena that are central to the discipline. Two of Lacan's papers—the one on the mirror stage and the one on aggressivity—do indeed try to do just that. My thesis, however, is that such necessity does not come from psychoanalytic experience but from the Hegelian framework underlying these papers.

I therefore propose to compare Lacan's theory of the mirror stage with the beginning statements of Hegel's discussion on the master-slave dialectic, and Lacan's theory of aggressivity with Hegel's discussion of the "Law of the Heart." I hope to show Lacan's dependence upon Hegel for providing the element of necessity required for the scientific status of his work, while at the same time drawing attention to the radical difference between Lacan and Hegel.

Lacan's Theory of the Mirror Stage and Hegel's Dialectic of Lordship and Bondage

Lacan's theory of the mirror stage is an attempt to answer the question, Why is it that the paranoid attacks his own ideal in the image of someone else? This question, as Muller and Richardson mention in their commentary on Lacan's *Écrits* (p. 329), was an important problem for Lacan as early as his doctoral thesis, *On Paranoia and Its Relationship to Personality.*

Lacan's answer makes use of two ideas. The first idea is that the human subject's emotional life must be radically transformed several times. These transformations occur because a number of frustrations are encountered—the process of weaning, the intrusion of siblings into the affective relationship with one's parents, and finally the Oedipus complex.[1] Each of these frustrations forces the subject to an emotional transformation that makes him accept more deeply the otherness of others. According to this theory, the absence of one or more of these transformations damages the extent to which the subject can relate to the other as other. Thus, the paranoiac can be understood to be a subject relating to another as if that other were his own self.

The second idea that Lacan needs in order to formulate his answer concerns the function of images or ideals: the human child does not experience his own unity until it *sees* that unity in the Gestalt of another human being or in the Gestalt of his own mirror image. Lacan claims that the human child becomes an "ego" only by means of this other: the mirror image. This theory explains Lacan's fondness for Rimbaud's aphorism, "'I' is 'another,'" which for Lacan means that "I" is based upon an "image borrowed from another."

Having seen the structural importance of the theory of the mirror stage in Lacan's thought, we can now look more closely at the theory of the mirror stage itself.

---

1. See Lacan's article on "La Famille." For a brief summary, see De Waelhens, *Schizophrenia*, pp. 123 ff. For a longer presentation, see De Waehlens, ch. 2, sects. 3 and 4.

Lacan's theory is an attempt to integrate several facts—scientific and cultural—and to make them intellectually understandable. The first scientific fact is this remarkable difference between a human baby and a baby chimpanzee: the chimpanzee at the age of about six to eight months has a manifestly greater problem-solving ability than the human baby; but it cannot grasp the meaning of the mirror image, while the human baby can. The chimpanzee tries to look behind the mirror to establish the reality of the image. When he establishes that nothing corresponds to the image, he loses interest in it. He is, therefore, unable to recognize himself in the mirror. The human baby on the contrary shows great interest, even excitement, in the image of himself that he sees in the mirror. Therefore, Lacan says, following others, he is able to recognize himself in the mirror image. Furthermore, Lacan stresses the fact that this recognition of the self in the mirror image has for the human baby a significant emotional meaning; there is a "flutter of jubilant activity" (*Écrits*, p. 1). Typical for the human baby, therefore, is not his problem-solving ability but his relation to his image.

The second scientific datum to be incorporated into the mirror-stage theory is the fact that for certain animals, seeing the Gestalt of their own species members has physiological consequences. An example is provided by L. Harrison Matthews' study, "Visual Stimulation and Ovulation in Pigeons" (1938–39), which proves that "the stimulus which causes ovulation in the pigeon is a *visual* one" (p. 558; my italics). A prior study by Harper had shown that "two female pigeons when confined together may both take to laying eggs" (p. 557), proving that the act of mating is not necessary for ovulation. Matthews' experiment then examined whether the necessary stimulus was visual, auditory, olfactory, or tactile, or a combination. He showed that ovulation occurs in female pigeons separated from either male or female pigeons by a sheet of glass, or even in a pigeon confined alone with a mirror, but does not occur in a pigeon that is in the same room with other birds but cannot see herself or other pigeons (p. 554). Matthews compares his results with those by two other researchers:

The *visual* stimulation here shown to exist in pigeons when confined with a single companion, or merely a mirror-image, is carried to a *higher level* in those birds which nest in colonies. Fraser Darling (1938) showed that a definite minimum number of pairs is a requisite in any breeding colony of certain species of birds that nest gregariously, in order to produce the threshold stimulus for ovulation. *Visual* stimulation has also been demonstrated in pigeons by Patel (1936), who showed that unless the male can *see* the female sitting on the eggs during incubation, he secretes no milk from the crop gland after the eggs are hatched. [pp. 559–60; my italics]

Lacan also mentions a study by Chauvin, which summarizes five years of research on the desert locust. As has been known since Uvarov, this locust can appear in a gregarious form and in a solitary form. The two differ in behavior, color, metabolic activity (oxygen and food intake), and physiology. Yet a transition from the solitary to the gregarious form is possible if the nymphs of a solitary locust are *in contact with members of their own species* during the early phases of their development. The age and sex of these other members is not relevant. However, they must be of the same or neighboring species. If they are members of a more distant species the transformation does not occur. According to Chauvin the contact must be *visual, tactile,* or by means of the locust's *antennae.* The mechanism of transformation of nymphs of a solitary locust into a gregarious locust explains the sporadic outbreak of the migratory locust.

Although Chauvin's study is more detailed, the study by Matthews provides more explicit support for the Lacanian thesis that seeing is the faculty which bridges the psychological and the physiological. Matthews' study confirms such a thesis for pigeons, but Chauvin's study of locusts, while it includes seeing as a transformation mechanism, does not exclude the sense of touch or the function of the antennae from this privileged position of bridge between psychology and physiology.

The third scientific fact to be incorporated into Lacan's theory of the mirror stage is transitivism in young children.[2] Lacan evokes this phenomenon when he writes: "The child who strikes another says that he has been struck; the child who sees another fall, cries" (*Écrits*, p. 19). The essence of the phenomenon is that young children identify so much with each other that they cannot distinguish between themselves and other children, and therefore ascribe to the other child what they themselves do to that child, and ascribe to themselves what is done to another.

The fourth fact to be incorporated into Lacan's theory of the mirror stage is man's fascination with dismemberment of the body, a fact from cultural history. According to Lacan, this fascination is present in such phenomena as "tattooing, incision, and circumcision." It is also present in man's dreams about "castration, mutilation, dismemberment, dislocation, evisceration, devouring, bursting open of the body," and in "the cruel refinement of the weapons" man has forged. Finally, it has been immortalized in the paintings of Hieronymus Bosch (*Écrits*, pp. 11, 12, 4).

The fifth and last scientific fact concerns the so-called prematurity of human birth. Lacan writes: "The anatomical incompleteness" of the human brain results in "signs of uneasiness and motor unco-ordination of the neo-natal months" (p. 4). He also approvingly quotes the label given by embryologists to this phenomenon: *foetalization.*

Lacan relates these facts to one another partly on an intentionally philosophical level. Thus, in his opening paragraph he writes about his theory of the mirror stage that "it is an experience that leads us to oppose any philosophy directly issuing from the *Cogito*" (*Écrits*, p. 1). Subsequently he talks about his theory as "an ontological structure of the human world" (p. 2) and "as a temporal dialectic that decisively projects the formation of the individual into history," which leads to "an alienating identity,

2. In his article on the mirror stage, Lacan mentions the work of Charlotte Bühler (p. 5). In his article on aggressivity he also mentions Elsa Köhler and the "Chicago School" which developed her ideas (p. 17), and finally also H. Wallon (p. 18).

which will mark with its rigid structure the subject's entire mental development" (p. 4). Finally, Lacan attacks Sartre's theory of negativity as incompatible with his theory of the mirror stage because Sartre still believes in the "self-sufficiency of consciousness, which, as one of its premises, links to the *méconnaissances* that constitute the ego, the illusion of autonomy to which it entrusts itself" (p. 6).

Lacan thus presents his view of man as an explicit antithesis to that of both Descartes and Sartre. He implicitly appeals to the Hegelian model when he attributes to the mirror stage the function of projecting the formation of the individual into history—that model being the master-slave dialectic, Hegel's attempt to explain why man is necessarily history-making. Before Hegel, both Fichte and Schelling had solved this problem by postulating at the dawn of mankind two human races, one rational and the other barbarous. Neither of these races had history; only their union made history and society possible. Hegel's analysis of the master-and-slave dialectic does not require the hypothesis of two human races, for it presents the inequality between men as emerging from within man himself.[3] The will to overcome this inequality then provides, for Hegel, the driving force for the making of history.

The history-creating possibility of this passage in Hegel's *Phenomenology* did not escape Kojève, the forceful commentator who introduced Hegel to a generation of French intellectuals, including Lacan. Kojève writes: "If man is nothing but his becoming, if his human existence in space is his existence in time or as time, if the revealed human reality is nothing but universal history, that history must be the history of the interaction between Mastery and Slavery: the historical 'dialectic' is the 'dialectic' of Master and Slave" (p. 9).

The above philosophical claims and the many explicit references to Hegel (e.g., *Écrits,* pp. 6, 26, 28) show both that Lacan is

---

3. For a convincing interpretation of Hegel's passage on "Lordship and Bondage," along the lines sketched above, see G. A. Kelly, "Notes on Hegel's 'Lordship and Bondage,'" particularly pp. 205 ff.

consciously creating a philosophical anthropology in his theory of the mirror stage and that he is dependent upon Hegel's dialectic of self-consciousness for his theoretical effort. The originality of Lacan's contribution lies in his attempt to tie Hegelian dialectical moves of the human subject, which resulted from a speculative understanding of history, to concrete scientific facts. This part of Lacan's effort puts his philosophical anthropology in radical opposition to the overall intent of Hegel's system.

The five facts that Lacan incorporates in his theory of the mirror stage are, as we saw, not all from the same scientific domain. Furthermore, some function as negative, others as positive facts. Foetalization and dismemberment function as negative facts. Foetalization is to be overcome and fantasies of dismemberment remind us that we can fall back to some undesirable state even though we might have overcome foetalization. Seeing, on the other hand, functions as the sense which can help man to overcome these negative facts. But how can seeing overcome these negative facts? It is here that it is important to stress that the five facts do not all belong to the same scientific domain.

Foetalization is an anatomico-physiological fact, whereas the fantasy of dismemberment is a psychological fact. Nevertheless, Lacan makes the fantasy of dismemberment function as a reminder that our bodily unity is a psychological achievement. He thus needs a transition between the two domains of the anatomico-physiological and of the psychological, and this is provided by the psychological function of seeing.

To these two domains of the physiological and the psychological Lacan must add the ontological domain, because he gives an ontological interpretation to some of the five facts he will incorporate in his theory of the mirror stage. Lacan interprets the foetalization of the human baby as constituting man as *lack*, and therefore as *to be* in the sense of *having to become*. But such an interpretation of a physiological fact is transposing by definition that fact into another domain, the domain of ontology of personhood. This will require that the fact which will remedy the foetalization—seeing—will itself receive an ontological interpretation. For Lacan, seeing produces an image capable of filling the lack which man is, and which will therefore almost imprison man by determining *unconsciously* the direction of his becoming. Man's essence, therefore, is not inside himself, as was suggested by the classic concept of the soul; man's essence is on the contrary located in something outside of himself:[4] the image that will guide his becoming. *I* am therefore *another*. If this is Lacan's ontological vision of man, then transitivism might become self-evident. It is the psychological manifestation of the ontological status of man.

The validity of Lacan's theory of the mirror stage will thus depend to a great extent upon the validity of the two ontological moves he makes: the foetalization of the human infant constituting man as lack, and the mirror image as another (or an image of oneself) so central to the self that that other becomes the master of one's own destiny. The second move shows a Hegelian influence, as we have seen. The first move shows a Heideggerian influence in that man is seen as *to be* or as *ecstatic*, which Lacan summarizes by his statement that man is lack. But these two ontological moves are neatly woven together by Lacan and are compatible in sharing a view of man in which man is radically dependent upon another, I want to concentrate on the second ontological move because it is this move which provides Lacan's theory of the mirror stage with its overall unity.

As already suggested, the basis of the second ontological move in Lacan's theory of the mirror stage can be found in the beginning paragraphs of Hegel's dialectic of self-consciousness, better known as the passage of the master-slave dialectic. I will quote these obscure passages and clarify them in order to make a comparison between Hegel and Lacan.

The beginning paragraph of "Lordship and Bondage" reads as follows: "Self-consciousness exists in itself and for itself in that, and by the fact that, it exists for another self-consciousness; that is to say, it *is* only by being acknowledged or 'recognized'" (*Phenomenology*, p. 229). Here Hegel rejects atomistic individualism as

---

4. This is central for Heidegger's ontology of the subject. For the relation between Heidegger and Lacan, see chapter 5, by Casey and Woody, section on Heidegger.

a correct description of the becoming of self-consciousness. Becoming self-conscious is, according to Hegel, not a product of the activity or of the will of an isolated individual. It is rather the *result* of an *intersubjective* relationship, of being acknowledged or recognized.

The second paragraph provides the arguments for the thesis stated in the first paragraph:

> Self-consciousness has before it another self-consciousness; it has come outside of itself. This has a double significance. First it has lost its own self, since it finds itself as an *other* being; secondly, it has thereby sublated that other, for it doesn't regard the other as essentially real, but sees its own self in the other.

The paragraph starts with a phenomenological description and continues with a logical analysis of that description. With the statement "Self-consciousness has before it another self-consciousness; it has come outside of itself," Hegel describes having before oneself another self-consciousness as involving an *act* whereby the first self-consciousness discovers in an external entity a quality of being that it has itself but that it was not yet consciously aware of. The first consciousness thereby *invests* in an external being qualities it has itself but is not yet fully aware of having. It is this *act of investment* that Hegel describes as the first consciousness "com[ing] outside of itself."

The remainder of the paragraph is a logical analysis of this phenomenological description. Hegel points out that to "come outside of" oneself in order to see another as a self-consciousness means two things. It means that the other is not constituted as *another* self-consciousness. The other is only constituted as a projection of the self-consciousness that the first consciousness has not yet become aware of in itself. In Hegel's words, the first self-consciousness "doesn't regard the other as essentially real, but sees its own self in the other." Hegel also points out that to "come outside" means that the first does not know itself, but on the contrary it has falsely discovered itself in another being and therefore has found itself as *another being*. As such, Hegel writes,

the first consciousness "has lost its own self." The logical analysis
of Hegel's phenomenological description points out that the full
constitution of another being as self-consciousness will involve
two steps. It will involve the step just described—that is, the constitution of the other as a self-consciousness. It will also, however,
involve the constitution of that self-consciousness as a self-consciousness that is *other* than the *own self*. Hegel's analysis seems to
stress that it is *false to believe that the second step can be reached without
the first step.* Both steps are necessary because the only way consciousness knows at first how to constitute another being as other
than itself is to constitute it as an object. Only when the other has
been constituted *first* as *another self-consciousness* can it afterward
be constituted as a *self-consciousness* that is *other than the own self*.

    The second paragraph serves as preparation for the ideas of
the next two paragraphs:

> It must cancel this other. To do so is the sublation of that
> first double meaning, and is therefore a second double
> meaning. First, it must set itself to sublate the other independ-
> ent being, in order thereby to become certain of itself as
> true being; secondly, it thereupon proceeds to sublate its
> own self, for this other is itself.
>
> This sublation in a double sense of its otherness in a double
> sense is at the same time a return in a double sense into its
> self. For, firstly, through sublation, it gets back itself, because
> it becomes one with itself/again through the cancelling of *its*
> otherness; but secondly, it likewise gives otherness back
> again to the other self-consciousness for it was aware of being
> in the other; it cancels this its own being in the other and then
> lets the other again go free. [pp. 229–30]

These paragraphs elaborate upon the second step required for
the full constitution of two self-consciousnesses. In the second
paragraph we learned that on the way to constituting itself as a
self-consciousness, the first consciousness constituted another
being as a self-consciousness that it itself actually was. In doing so,
the first self-consciousness did not constitute a *real other*, and it did
not discover its *own self*. On the contrary, the first consciousness

discovered itself *in and as* another self-consciousness. There is therefore otherness in the heart of self-consciousness. But a self is not the otherness that it needs as a means to discover or to constitute itself as a self-consciousness. In order, therefore, to become really a *self*-consciousness, consciousness will have to *destroy that otherness in the heart of self-consciousness.* Only in this way can the first consciousness overcome the loss of self discussed in the second paragraph.

In the process of constituting a real self-awareness by destroying the otherness in its own heart, consciousness differentiates between the self-consciousness it is and the self-consciousness the other is. It thereby sees the other as *other* rather than as *another self.*

These opening paragraphs of Hegel's "Lordship and Bondage" thus establish that the transition from consciousness to self-consciousness requires an *intermediate step* in which *a first consciousness discovers itself in another self-consciousness.* This intermediate step is alienating and must be overcome. Given the logical necessity of this intermediate step, we can now say that the ontological description of the process of becoming a self-consciousness *includes necessarily* a relation to another in whom I discover myself as a self-consciousness.

Lacan takes over the essence of Hegel's ontology of self-consciousness, while at the same time transforming it enough to be applicable to the five facts mentioned earlier. Like Hegel, Lacan maintains that the subject needs another in order to become a subject. Lacan, however, restates Hegel's ontology of self-consciousness as follows: at six months of age the human subject gives itself objectivity and permanence by *seeing* itself in the Gestalt of another or even in the Gestalt of its own mirror image. It then invests this Gestalt libidinally, giving rise to the stage called *primary narcissism.*

In both cases the *structure* of the ontological description of the self is the same. Lacan does not follow Hegel in stressing the *logical necessity* of an *intermediate step* in the transition from consciousness to self-consciousness. Nevertheless, the theory of the mirror stage is presented as a necessary part of the ontology of the human subject (*Écrits*, p. 2). Lacan is therefore dependent upon the Hegelian analysis of self-consciousness in order to give the mirror stage its necessity. Lacan's dependence upon Hegel is also obvious when one analyzes the relation of transitivism to the mirror stage. The latter theory points to the apprehension of the Gestalt of another's body as necessary in order for the human subject to be able to appropriate and to unify its own body. It explains how the Gestalt of another is instrumental for the appropriation of one's own body. If therefore offers an explanation of why one child starts making exactly the same gestures as another. But this theory does not immediately explain why one child should cry when another child falls. To do so one needs the Hegelian idea that consciousness "sees *its own self* in the other." In Lacan one self relates to the Gestalt of another; in Hegel, however, a self relates to *another self* because the first self discovers itself in the other as *self-consciousness*. The latter intersubjective relation has a depth which allows us to understand why one child cries when another falls. Under Lacan's more restricted theory we would expect that when one child falls the other child would fear that it too will fall, because this child's body experience is dominated by the Gestalt of the other. We expect such a child *to fear, not to cry.*

Thus, notwithstanding the dependence of Lacan's theory of the mirror stage upon Hegel's dialectic of self-consciousness, we should not overlook the difference between Hegel's analysis and Lacan's theory.

A first difference between Hegel's dialectic of self-consciousness and Lacan's dialectic of the mirror stage concerns the status of the subject before it enters the dialectic. In Hegel we have a consciousness that has discovered its own role in knowing the world. It lacks only the method needed to find out who it is. In Lacan we have a subject who is ill at ease with himself, who is uncoordinated, who is anatomically incomplete, and who experiences his movements as turbulence (*Écrits*, pp. 3–4). By means of the mirror stage the subject is offered an idealized unity that he does not have at that moment. By means of the Gestalt of another, Lacan's subject is not just *finding out* who he is but rather is *creating* himself as what he is not yet but in some sense should become. What is hereby created, therefore, is not a self-consciousness but rather an organizing matrix, a statue (p. 2), and this organizing matrix Lacan calls "I."

A second difference between the Hegelian and the Lacanian dialectic is in their result. In Hegel the dialectic of self-consciousness leads consciousness to become aware of itself as the negative of objectivity. In a further moment of the dialectic, however, self-consciousness will become humble because of its fear of death. It thereby is willing to give a positive function to the other than itself—that is, objectivity (life, the body, etc.). Thus, the dialectic in Hegel allows consciousness to see what the dialectic is about because it is consciousness itself that is invited to give meaning to the other than the self. In Lacan the dialectic of the mirror stage results in the creation of an idealized organizing matrix that the subject is not, but that the subject projects itself as becoming. That Gestalt, that *idealized statue,* has a content which the subject appropriates without a conscious justification. Contrary to Hegel's dialectic, the Lacanian dialectic of the mirror stage does not assign consciousness a crucial role in bringing about the dialectic move. Instead, Lacan has assigned this crucial role to the influence upon the child of the structural signifiers: the Gestalt of another, and the name-of-the-father; the latter signifier is analyzed in Lacan's article on psychosis (*Écrits,* pp. 179–225).

A third difference between the Hegelian and Lacanian dialectics is their focus. In Hegel the dialectic is the process whereby consciousness becomes aware of what it is and then affirms its discovery in reality. It discovers itself first of all as *negativity.* In Lacan the dialectic is about the subject conquering its body as an exteriority. That body has a visual unity that the interior experience of the same body does not have. The mirror stage is therefore an instrument to synthesize the subject as *spatiality.*

These three differences are dictated by Lacan's concern with the scientific facts previously mentioned—in particular, the physiological consequences of seeing the image of one's own Gestalt or the Gestalt of members of one's species, and the foetalization phenomenon. The differences locate the Lacanian dialectic more at the bodily level than at the conscious level. The Lacanian dialectic also implies that in the mirror stage a statue, a content that the subject does not consciously understand, gets hold of the subject. Inasmuch as Lacan claims that the synthesis achieved in the mirror stage is a foundation, a basis for further syntheses (or identifications), Lacan's theory presents us with a view of man in which an unconscious, alien identity is the basis of any further psychological development. Within such a framework, the Hegelian dream of conscious self-possession is radically impossible.

There is another possible comparison with Hegel in the function of aggressivity that Lacan hints at in his paper (*Écrits*, p. 6). This aggressivity could be related to the life-and-death struggle described in Hegel's dialectic of self-consciousness. Lacan makes this problem the object of a separate article, though, and I shall also devote a separate discussion to this theme.

Lacan's Theory of Aggressivity and Hegel's Passage on the Law of the Heart

I wish to argue briefly that the aggressivity present in the life-and-death struggle between the two consciousnesses who will become the master and the slave can illustrate only one of the forms of aggressivity that Lacan's theory deals with. I believe that the passage on the "Law of the Heart" illustrates Lacan's main point in his theory of aggressivity.

The main point of Lacan's theory of aggressivity is that aggressivity is a defensive strategy used when the loss of an ideal threatens the unity of the self. This is related to the theory of the mirror stage, in which an idealized image provides the subject with a unity that it does not have in fact but that it gives itself by means of an idealized project.

The aggressivity involved in the master-slave dialectic is not defensive or repressive. On the contrary, the life-and-death struggle has a very positive function. It is the only way by which the two consciousnesses can prove the truth of their feelings that as consciousnesses they are not tied to objectivity. Moreover, the life-and-death struggle in Hegel's dialectic is an attack on the other which involves a risk of the self, rendering it a progressive and not a regressive move at this point of the *Phenomenology*. The attack on the other seems consonant with Lacan. However, a careful study of Hegel's text demonstrates that Hegel does not interpret the attack of a consciousness on another consciousness in the Lacanian sense. The purpose of the struggle is *not* to destroy the self in the other (one's ideal in the image of someone else) but to destroy the otherness in the other self. It is the otherness in the other self that is attacked in the master-slave dialectic and not the *self* in the other.[5]

The master-slave dialectic can, however, be a useful point of comparison with respect to a second, though less important, form of aggressivity talked about by Lacan. In the first part of his essay (particularly in the presentation of the second thesis), Lacan mentions the aggressivity exercised by the person serving as model or image for the subject of the mirror stage. Lacan's strategy at this point of the essay seems to be to draw attention to the fact that the relation between the subject and his image has a link with aggressivity from the beginning. According to that quick hint of Lacan's (*Écrits*, pp. 10–11), the subject has not tied himself down to an image purely spontaneously but also because of the threat of the model itself. The idea that threat is essential if education is to be effective, or if a person is to be able to live up to the standards of an ideal, is an idea cherished by Hegel. Hegel writes in his *Philosophy of Right*:

> Similarly, the right of the parents over the wishes of their children is determined by the object in view—discipline and education. The punishment of children does not aim at justice as such; the aim is more subjective and moral in character, i.e., to deter them from exercising a freedom still in the toils of nature and to lift the universal into their consciousness and will. [p. 117]

5. *Phenomenology:* "the other's reality is presented to the former as an external other, as outside itself; it must cancel that externality" (p. 233). "It must cancel this other. . . . First, it must set itself to sublate the other independent being, in order thereby to become certain of itself as true being" (p. 229).

The necessary fear of a model is expressed as part of a systematic analysis of consciousness's experience of itself at the end of the passage on the master-slave dialectic, where Hegel writes: "Without the discipline of service and obedience, fear remains formal and does not spread over the whole known reality of existence" (*Phenomenology*, p. 239). Thus the fear of death is not productive of a further development of consciousness unless the *threat of the master* uses that fear to impose on the slave the discipline required to fulfill his commands. It is in trying to fulfill these commands that the slave deals with his own desires. He is forced to work and develop skills. And about work Hegel writes: "Labour, on the other hand, is desire restrained and checked, evanescence delayed and postponed, in other words, labour shapes and fashions the thing" (p. 238). The slave can achieve such a constructive mastery of his own desires only by means of a *threat* by another. Furthermore, we know that this other (the master) functions as the "ideal ego" for the slave.[6] Lacan's reference to the "severe parent" or the "image of the Punisher" can therefore be taken to be more than a reference to a fact. It can be taken by means of the Hegelian dialectic to be a reference to a *necessity of consciousness*.[7]

The passage on the "Law of the Heart," which can clarify the other and more important aspect of Lacan's theory of aggressivity, is part of the third great movement in the *Phenomenology*. The first movement describes the enrichment of consciousness when it relates to objects. Consciousness discovers that it cannot know the objects by senses only; it needs to use words (perception) and thoughts (scientific understanding). The second movement describes the adventures of consciousness encountering another consciousness and thereby becoming self-consciousness. As we have seen, Hegel believes that the crucial concern of two con-

---

6. *Phenomenology:* "The master is taken to be the essential reality for the state of bondage" (p. 237). "In the master, the bondsman feels self-existence to be something external, an objective fact" (p. 239). "He sees in the master . . . self-existence as a real mode of consciousness" (p. 241).

7. Muller and Richardson see in this transition a big problem for Lacan (pp. 46–47). But if one situates Lacan's thought also within Hegel's philosophy then the transition can be said to be there from the start, without having to be justified.

sciousnesses meeting each other is not knowledge but recognition; it is possible to interpret the movement describing the adventures of self-consciousness as the description of the different strategies that self-consciousness can adopt to gain recognition. The third movement describes the experience of an enriched self-consciousness. It is a self-consciousness which has become certain of itself and is therefore not directly or immediately concerned with recognition. It is a self-consciousness which has discovered that it possesses reason. It is a self-consciousness which trusts that in and through reason it can *know the other than itself*, it can *know the world*.

At first such a rational self-consciousness is puzzled by the objective world. It learns, however, that knowledge of the outside world does not inform itself about the secret most dear to it—that is, itself. Rational self-consciousness therefore makes the move of actively relating self-consciousness to the outside world. The first method is relating self-consciousness' desire (pleasure) to the outside world. That outside world can be either the laws of nature or the rules of social etiquette. Both appear to consciousness as an external imposition, but given that self-consciousness is rational, it should have provided the norm of all rules rather than having them imposed from without.

Out of this experience emerges the sentimentalism of the romantic movement, which takes the principle of reason in man as the norm for societal arrangements. The principle of reason is that, by thinking, I as individual have access to the universal rules by which nature and society ought to be ordered. Applied to the social order the principle of reason means that I as rational individual have access to these universal rules by means of my heart, which represents the heart of all men. It is this move of *rational individual self-consciousness* which allows Hegel to explain by the same principle the emergence of natural science and the romantic movement. Both are the result of the principle of subjectivity, which emerged, according to Hegel, as a central principle of modern times: consciousness takes itself to have the point of view from which to legislate the outside world. When the outside world is nature, the legislating takes the form of *description* by means of natural laws; when the outside world is the social order, the legislating takes the form of *prescription*.

Let us now look at the passage on the "Law of the Heart" and the function of aggressivity in it. The experience that gives rise to the project of romantic sentimentalism is that the laws of nature or the rules of etiquette are a barrier to the enjoyment of self-consciousness. The project thus becomes opposition to these barriers on rational grounds or by means of a justification typical for modern times. *The barrier that I experience is assumed to be a barrier experienced by all.* I can thus project an alternative order that on the same principle *should be acceptable to all.* Thus, social reform can be experienced by the romantic person as *a reform for the "welfare of mankind"* (*Phenomenology*, p. 392).

The problem with this project is that all reforms will involve the presentation of new rules that will appear as *new barriers.* Because of these new barriers the romantic reformer must ultimately be angry unless he can experience them as *his* barriers, and see that there are barriers that he finds rational. The angry reformer remains naive. If he takes the second road he has become a member of a social order (p. 394). He has accepted that there must be rules in any social order and that such rules are at some times a barrier to one's satisfaction. He is, however, at this point *capable only of accepting the rules that he himself is thinking.* Indeed, the purpose of the romantic reformer was not to put forth societal rules but to have societal rules which the heart of man could identify with. This whole enterprise was built on the belief that it is possible to have *laws that are identical with the wishes of the heart.* And the romantic reformer takes the wishes of *his* heart to be normative for the wishes of *all* hearts.

The crucial turn in the dialectic of the law of the heart occurs when Hegel points out that other people find in the laws espoused by the romantic reformer not the law of *their* hearts but the law of *another* heart. Thus, remarks Hegel, the romantic reformer believes that something particular (the *law* of *his* heart) has universal validity, whereas others see the proposals of the romantic reformer for what they are—*a particular law imposed on them.* And just as the romantic reformer opposed societal laws imposed on him, so the others oppose the proposal of the romantic reformer.

The romantic reformer thus faces two problems. First, he must be able to accept that there must be societal laws. But even if he proposes laws, his heart does not feel comfortable with any law. Second, in making the attempt to reconcile himself with the *law* of *his* heart, he faces the problem that *others will reject his law for the same reasons that he started his romantic reforms.*

The fact that consciousness experiences societal laws as *necessary* but that this consciousness as particular consciousness finds societal laws in general worthy of rejection is for Hegel sufficient reason to conclude that we are faced here with a consciousness that is perverse. It is the craziness, the madness of consciousness. *How can consciousness deal with this, its own essential madness?* Hegel's answer is worth quoting:

> The heart throb for the welfare of mankind passes therefore into the rage of fanatic self-conceit, into the fury of consciousness to preserve itself from destruction; and to do so by casting out of its life the perversion which it really is, and by straining to regard and to express that perversion as something else. The universal ordinance and law it, therefore, now speaks of as an utter distortion of the law of its heart and of its happiness, a perversion invented by fanatical priests, by riotous, revelling despots and their minions, who seek to indemnify themselves for their own degradation by degrading and oppressing in their turn—a distortion practiced to the nameless misery of deluded mankind. [*Phenomenology*, p. 391]

Consciousness is perverted consciousness when it requires that societal rules be the direct expression of the wishes of the individual's heart. Hegel's dialectic shows that the perversion of such a consciousness is a *necessary* one. *Perverted consciousness defends itself against this experience of its own perversion by projecting it onto another.* It is in the other(s) that it attacks its own perversion.

At least three elements of Lacan's theory of aggressivity remind us of Hegel's dialectic of the Law of the Heart. First, just as Hegel presupposes that the romantic reformer is dominated by the will to reform social reality according to the wishes of his heart, so Lacan claims that man has a "passionate desire . . . to impress his image in reality" (*Écrits,* p. 22).

In the rest of the text Lacan goes so far as to say that the rational will which *restricts* itself to rational transformation of the world is to be related to that furious passion of man that wants to change the world in order to see the world give testimony to its own image. He calls that furious passion "the obscure basis of the rational mediations of the will" (p. 22).

Second, just as Hegel demonstrates that it is typical for the romantic reformer to situate himself in the societal reality in such a way that he and others are mortal enemies, so Lacan claims that man's narcissistic identification with his image constitutes man as aggressive competitor with other men (p. 23). Lacan attaches great importance to this development of man into aggressive competitor. He describes it in his theory as a *necessary moment.* He even gives it a status that rivals the importance of his theory of the mirror stage and of Freud's Oedipus complex. To this moment he has given the name "Intrusion complex." As early as his 1938 article on the family,[8] Lacan had used this element of his theory to elevate the fact of sibling rivalry from a *deplorable fact* into a *necessary moment* in the constitution of the self.

Third, just as Hegel describes the romantic reformer as attacking in the other his own perversion, so Lacan claims that the *aggressivity* of the paranoiac has the dual purpose of projecting something unacceptable in him onto another and of attacking it in that other. Indeed, he writes: "And the two moments, when the subject denies himself and when he charges the other, become confused, and one discovers in him that paranoiac structure of the ego" (p. 20). In order to reinforce this view of the paranoiac, Lacan refers to Freud's study on Judge Schreber. In that study Freud relates paranoia to homosexuality and claims that the paranoiac tries to *deny* the proposition "*I* (a man) *love him*

---

8. Lacan, "La Famille," pp. 840.8–.11. For a brief English version of the main ideas of Lacan's "Intrusion complex," see De Waelhens, pp. 76–79, "The Sibling or the Incarnated Mirror-Image."

(a man)" by denying either one of the elements of that sentence or the whole sentence. Furthermore, Freud points out that the paranoiac projects onto another his own denied action (1911, p. 63).

This similarity between Hegel and Lacan is not accidental. Lacan himself stresses the fact that his conception of paranoiac delusion is identical to the delusion of Hegel's misanthropic beautiful soul.[9] In that same passage Lacan refers to Freud, too, thereby relating his own conclusion to crucial passages in two of his intellectual mentors:

> And the two moments, when the subject denies himself and when he charges the other, become confused, and one discovers in him that paranoiac structure of the ego that finds its analogue in the fundamental negations described by Freud as the three delusions of jealousy, erotomania, and interpretation. It is the especial delusion of the misanthropic *'belle âme'* [beautiful soul], throwing back on to the world the disorder of which his being is composed. [p. 20]

We should not, however, overlook the differences between Lacan's and Hegel's views of aggressivity. An obvious difference is that the two authors situate aggressivity in different domains. Hegel locates the unavoidability of aggressivity in the *social domain*. Aggressivity becomes unavoidable because the individual remains individualistic and requires that for any societal rule to be acceptable, it must conform to the wishes of his *own* heart.[10] Lacan, on the contrary, situates the aggressivity in *the spatial dimension* of man. For Lacan, my body as my subjective space is not available to me at the start. The act of appropriating my body as my space is done by means of a psychological act of identifying with an idealized image. Given that the subject is not this ide-

9. Lacan, *Écrits*, p. 20. "Misanthropic beautiful soul" is a metaphoric reference for consciousness as Hegel describes it in the "Law of the Heart." It should not be confused with the passage on the "Beautiful Soul." Hegel, *Phenomenology*, pp. 390–400, 642–79, respectively.

10. The individualistic point of view is overcome as soon as consciousness reaches the level of Spirit (p. 451). The passage of the "Law of the Heart" is one of the last passages before the one on Spirit.

alized image, Lacan claims that the bodily unity can be achieved only by means of imposing on others and the world that idealized self-image. This is the hidden aggressivity mentioned by Lacan, which becomes open aggressivity when that idealized image is threatened.

A second difference between Hegel's and Lacan's views on aggressivity is the way in which both see the solution to this aggressivity. For Hegel, the solution comes when the individual is able to give up the individualistic point of view and to identify with the point of view of the spirit (i.e., truth having a societal and objective point of view). Hegel defines this point of view as follows:

> Spirit is the self of the actual consciousness to which spirit stands opposed, or rather which appears over against itself, as an objective actual world that has lost, however, all sense of strangeness for the self, just as the self has lost all sense of having a dependent or independent existence by itself, cut off and separated from that world. [*Phenomenology*, p. 458]

For Lacan, the solution lies in the Oedipus complex: "Thus the Oedipal identification is that by which the subject transcends the aggressivity that is constitutive of the primary subjective individuation" (*Écrits*, p. 23). In the Oedipus complex, the subject creates an ego ideal on the basis of the image of the father. About the ego ideal, Lacan writes,

> What concerns us here is the function that I shall call the pacifying function of the ego ideal, the connexion between its libidinal normativity and a cultural normativity bound up from the dawn of history with the *imago* of the father. [p. 22]

Both differences indicate that Lacan takes a *more particularized* point of view than Hegel. For Hegel the aggressivity of the romantic reformer is connected with a lack of rationality in that consciousness. This form of aggressivity is then also irrational. Once rationality has been broadened and has reached the point of view of Spirit, then aggressivity is rational in the specific sense that it is connected with *rational goals*. Thus, for Hegel the aggressivity demanded by the state in the case of war is a rational form of aggressivity because it subordinates individualistic and particularistic interests to the interest of the state, interpreted by Hegel as the universal. For Lacan, however, the problem of aggressivity is connected with the very way in which man must appropriate the spatiality of his being. For Lacan, aggressivity is therefore coextensive with man's appropriation of himself as a unified body.[11] According to Lacan's theory, aggressivity must therefore be an omnipresent phenomenon for the individual as embodied subject. We find a confirmation of that in his reference to the aggressivity present in all philanthropic activity (p. 13).

Conclusion

I have argued that the logical necessity which Lacan presents as part of his theory of the mirror stage and of his theory of aggressivity is dependent upon two separate moves in Hegel's *Phenomenology*. The theory of the mirror stage includes the thesis that another than the self is necessary for the constitution of the self. The beginning pages of "Lordship and Bondage" establish that the transition from consciousness to self-consciousness requires an *intermediate step* in which a first consciousness discovers *itself* in *another self-consciousness*.

Lacan's theory of aggression includes the thesis that aggressivity is an attack upon the self in another. Hegel's passages in "The Law of the Heart" present us with a consciousness (the romantic reformer) which on the one hand incorporates the principle of modern times that the individual has in reason *the* correct principle to discover the rules of reality, and on the other hand emotionally identifies the wishes of its own heart with those of the hearts of others. This consciousness experiences itself as perverse because in executing its project it necessarily does the opposite of what it intends. It can deal with this perversion because it identifies its own heart with the hearts of others. This identity is thus the origin of and the solution for its perversion. Indeed, it can

11. Lacan, *Écrits*, p. 28: "the extent to which the fear of death . . . is psychologically subordinate to the narcissistic fear of damage to one's own body."

condemn and attempt to destroy in the other what went wrong in its own heart. An attack upon the self in the other is therefore a possibility and a necessity, because consciousness is engaged with others in the world, while lacking initially the distinction between its own heart and the heart of others.

In this chapter I also drew attention to some radical differences between Lacan's theories and the passages in Hegel. In the mirror stage we are dealing not with another self but with the Gestalt of another as constitutive of the self. In Lacan's theory of aggressivity we are not in the presence of a consciousness that lacks a distinction. We are in the presence of an embodied consciousness that can maintain its unity (including its bodily unity) only by means of an ideal which it is not. It therefore needs to impose this ideal on the others. In both cases, therefore, Lacan analyzes a bodily self rather than a consciousness.

What, then, is the subject of Lacan? Even though he uses Hegelian moves in the explanation of his view of the subject, Lacan's subject is not a Hegelian consciousness. The importance given to the bodily element will allow Lacan to introduce in his concept of a subject the idea of radical finitude. He even has at his disposal Heidegger's philosophy in order to do so. Given the openness of Heidegger's philosophy to the crucial function of language, we now see how linguistics can be incorporated in Lacan's philosophical anthropology. It is this aspect of Lacan's theory of the subject which is masterfully explained in chapter 4 of this volume, by William Richardson. However, by stressing almost exclusively the Heideggerian influence in Lacan, Richardson fails to present Lacan's subject as an emotional force, which will in its history encounter radical frustration (weaning, intrusion, castration). This history has logical necessity, as De Waelhens' readings of Lacan have demonstrated (*Schizophrenia*, ch. 2, sects. 3, 4). De Waelhens' reading is dependent on the early Lacan found in his article on the family. It is a reading of Lacan that is compatible with Lacan's own claim of a return to Freud, since it is in Freud that we find the idea of the subject as libido, with a normative development from autoeroticism through narcissism to heterosexuality. Too much stress on the Heideggerian influence in Lacan makes us lose sight of the developmental norms through which the Lacanian subject unfolds.

Finally, I should remark that the "Other" in Lacan is indeed different from Freud's "other scène," as Antoine Vergote so clearly demonstrates in chapter 9. A crucial difference is the fact that Lacan's "Other" has a claim to truth that is more radical than Freud's "other scène." Lacan writes that the "Other" is "the locus from which the question of his existence may be presented to him" (*Écrits*, p. 194). It would be useful to pursue the Hegelian influence in Lacan's treatment of the concept of the "Other," given that Hegel himself locates the point of view of the truth in the subject's ability to see himself as a relation with the Other (the societal norms and truths) of the self (*Phenomenology*, pp. 457–61).

REFERENCES

Chauvin, R. "Contribution à l'étude physiologique du criquet pélerin et du determinism des phénomènes grégaires." *Annales de la Societé entomologique de France* 110 (1941): 133–272.
De Waelhens, A. *Schizophrenia*. Pittsburgh: Duquesne University Press, 1978.
Freud, S. "Psycho-Analytic Notes on an Autobiographical Account of a Case of Paranoia" (1911). *Standard Edition of the Complete Psychological Works*, vol. 12. London: Hogarth, 1958.
Hegel, G.W.F. *The Phenomenology of Mind*. Translated by J. B. Baillie. New York: Humanities Press, 1980.
———. *Philosophy of Right*. Translated by T. M. Knox. New York: Oxford University Press, 1967.
Kelly, G. A. "Notes on Hegel's 'Lordship and Bondage.'" In A. MacIntyre, ed., *Hegel*. New York: Doubleday, 1972.
Kojève, A. *Introduction to the Reading of Hegel* (1947). Lectures on *The Phenomenology of Spirit*, assembled by R. Queneau. Edited by A. Bloom. Translated by J. H. Nichols, Jr. New York: Basic Books, 1969.
Lacan, J. *Écrits: A Selection*. Translated by A. Sheridan. New York: Norton, 1977.
———. "La Famille," which includes two separate but related articles, "Le complexe, facteur concret du lien psychologique familiale," pp.

840.5–840.16; "Les complexes familiaux en pathologie," pp. 841.1–842.8, in *Encyclopédie Française*. Vol. 8. Paris: Larousse, 1938.

Matthews, L. H. "Visual Stimulation and Ovulation in Pigeons." *Proceedings of the Royal Society of London, Series B 126* (1938–39): 557–60.

Muller, J. P., and Richardson, W. J. *Lacan and Language: A Reader's Guide to Écrits*. New York: International Universities Press, 1982.

7

Psychoanalysis and the Being-question

WILLIAM J. RICHARDSON

"Of all the undertakings that have been proposed in this century, that of the psychoanalyst is perhaps the loftiest, because his task is to act in our time as a mediator between the man of care [i.e., human being according to Heidegger] and the subject of absolute knowledge [i.e., human being according to Hegel]" (Lacan, 1977, p. 105/321, slightly emended).[1] Lofty undertaking, indeed—perhaps futile—but the vastness of the challenge suggests both the audacity of Lacan's own endeavor and the depth of the sources from which he derives his inspiration. To be sure, there were other philosophical influences on him besides Heidegger and Hegel—over the course of the years he turned to thinkers from Heraclitus to Merleau-Ponty—but it was these two Germans in particular who marked him most deeply, and their influence remained even after he ceased to refer to them.

Whether or not the mediation suggested in Lacan's remark is ultimately feasible, the fact remains that any attempt to understand his thought in terms of its philosophical underpinnings must begin by assessing separately the influence of each of these two thinkers on him in turn. It is to the first of these tasks that I address myself here, attempting to understand (in part, at least) what made Heidegger's thought so attractive to Lacan and what light this thought may throw upon Lacan's own innovative insight.

---

1 For any foreign work cited, where an English translation exists, I refer first to the pagination in the English text, then to its equivalent in the original. Occasionally these translations have been slightly emended. Where no published translation exists, texts have been translated by the author.

What that innovative insight was is now a commonplace: "The unconscious [Freud's great discovery] is structured like a language." How this unconscious—"that part of the concrete discourse, in so far as it is transindividual, that is not at the disposition of the subject in re-establishing the continuity of his conscious discourse" (1977, p. 49/258, slightly emended)—is to be conceived according to Lacan has been described in some detail in chapter 4 of this volume. His essential assertion is that the unconscious is Other than the subject. As such, it is somehow ultimate, for we are told that there is "no Other of the Other" (1977, p. 311/813), meaning that there is no metalanguage, no more fundamental system of signifiers on which the symbolic order is grounded.

No metalanguage, then. Yet Lacan often speaks of the Other in terms of Being.[2] "The force [of the unconscious] comes from the truth and in the dimension of Being: *Kern unseres Wesens* are Freud's own words" (1977, p. 116/518). And again, "The neurosis is a question that Being poses for a subject. . . . The 'Being' referred to is that which appears in a lightning moment in the void of the verb 'to be'" (1977, p. 168/520). Certainly the Heideggerian tone is evident.

But there is better evidence still. In the seminar of 1955, we find the following:

> In a dream there is always a point that is absolutely ungraspable, Freud tells us, and it belongs to the domain of the unknown—he calls it the navel (*Nabel: ombilic*) of the dream. We do not underline these things in his text because we probably imagine that it is [just] poetry. No, indeed. It means that there is a point that is not graspable in the phenomenon, the point of the emergence of the relation of the subject to the symbolic. What I call Being is this last word that is not accessible to us, certainly, in the scientific attitude but the direction of which is indicated in the phenomenon of our experience. [1954–55, p. 130]

2. I capitalize the word "Being" when I understand it to stand for Heidegger's *Sein,* and leave it in lower case for Heidegger's *Seiendes,* i.e., "that-which-is" or "entity."

This suggests that Being for Lacan, "the point of emergence of the relation of the subject to the symbolic," is more radical than the symbolic order as Lévi-Strauss conceived it—more radical, too, than the human subject as Lacan conceives it. In a similar tone, we read later in the same seminar:

> The fundamental relationship of man to this symbolic order is quite precisely that which founds the symbolic order itself—the relation of non-Being to Being. . . . The end of the symbolic process is that non-Being come to be (*vienne à être*), and this because it has come into words (*a parlé*). [1954–55, p. 354]

What this might mean we infer from Lacan's frequent allusion to the famous *fort-da* experience as described by Freud (1920, pp. 14–15). In his mother's absence, the child in question would throw a reel into a curtained cot, making it disappear. As he did so, he uttered the sound "o-o-o-o," which Freud surmised was the child's equivalent of the German word *fort,* or "away." When he pulled the reel out of the cot, he would utter "*da*" ("here"). By uttering these two phonemes, the child was playing a game of separation and return. For Lacan, the significance of this little game had less to do with the "renunciation of instinctual satisfaction" experienced in the mother's absence than with the child's burgeoning realization of the power of speech to make what is absent become present through language (1977, p. 103/319). Thus, although the "pure function [of the symbolic order] is manifested in a thousand ways in human life, [this] function is [reducible to] terms of presence and absence, of Being (*être*) and Non-being (*non-être*)" (1954–55, p. 367).

In the early sixties, apparently beginning with the seminar on "Identification" in 1961–62, Lacan's interest began to shift toward a greater emphasis on formalism and mathematics, and in 1964 he refers to his former appeal to Heidegger as a "propaedeutic reference" only (1964, p. 18/22). Nonetheless, he admits that it is an "ontological function that is at stake in this gap (*béance*) by which [he] felt obliged to introduce the function of the unconscious" (1964, p. 29/31). Moreover, this gap opens up and closes intermittently—a kind of "pulsating function" (1964, p. 43/44), essentially "evasive," that can be diserned in a structure that is "temporal" in a way that he claims "up to now has never been articulated as such" (1964, p. 32/33). An ontological function that is "evasive" and essentially "temporal" in nature retains the Heideggerian ring.

In 1972, in his seminar *Encore*, Lacan was in the full flush of his formalism. There must be a complete "rupture," he says, with anything that smacks of philosophy. "Mathematical formalism is our aim, our ideal" (1972–73, p. 108). There is evident hostility to the notion of "Being." "There is no metalanguage," he insists. "When I say that, that means apparently, no language of Being. But is there Being? . . . Being is, as they say, and Non-being is not. . . . This Being can be supposed only for certain words—individual, for example, or substance" (1972–73, p. 107). What he insists upon here, then, is that however one understands the ultimate nature of language, it cannot be grounded in something "subsistent in itself, by itself, all alone, as the language of Being" (1972–73, p. 108)—he seems to mean some kind of absolute thing-in-itself, above, beyond, or behind the symbolic order. "It is thus that the symbolic is not confused—far from it—with Being, but subsists as the existence of speaking [as such] (*comme existence du dire*)" (1972–73, p. 108). He seems to be saying, then, that there is no Other of the Other, not even Being itself—if, that is, Being be conceived as some ontic absolute transcendent to the symbolic order as such. But is this indeed the case? Let us turn to Heidegger to see if his reflection on the matter can be of help.

The general lines of Heidegger's development are by now quite clear. It all began in 1907 when, at the age of eighteen, he came upon Brentano's doctoral dissertation, "The Manifold Sense of 'being' in Aristotle," where "being" is the Greek *on* (*Seiendes*):

> On the title page of his work, Brentano quotes Aristotle's phrase, *to on legetai pollachōs*. I translate: "'a being' [entity] becomes manifest, i.e., with regard to its Being, in many ways." Latent in this phrase is the *question* that determines the way of my thought: What is the pervasive, simple, unified

determination of Being that permeates all of its possible meanings? [1974, p. x]

It was twenty years later that the major work, *Being and Time* (1927), appeared.

By way of résumé, we may say that there have been three generations of interpreters of that work—or at least three levels of interpretation. The first generation focused on *Being and Time* itself and the relatively few other works of the period. The best known of these interpretations is that of Alphonse de Waelhens, *The Philosophy of Martin Heidegger* (1942). But after World War II, Heidegger published a number of other works that reveal a different style, a different emphasis from that of *Being and Time*— some said a different philosophy, born of the failure of the early effort. Most characteristic of this period was a focus on Being rather than on man (*Dasein*). This period culminated in 1962 with the lecture "Time and Being," where Heidegger tried to "think Being without beings" (1972, p. 2/2) and proposed as ultimate key to the problem the notion of *Ereignis*, "event of appropriation." His critics maintained that this sort of theorizing either became a kind of mysticism that was no longer philosophy or else relapsed into a hypostasizing of Being that revealed itself and concealed itself in peekaboo fashion to man.

The second generation of interpreters focused on the publications of the fifties, usually showing the unity of (therefore continuity between) the two periods. In effect, some tried to argue that the later period was a "re-trieve" (*Wiederholung*) of the unsaid of the earlier period and postulated that there was a deeper source of unity still to be explored, to which was given the name of the "Ur-Heidegger" (Richardson, 1974, p. 632).

Now, more than twenty years later, there is another generation of interpreters who explore this "Ur-Heidegger"—that is, the Heidegger of the incubation years of *Being and Time,* accessible now thanks to the gradual publication of the collected works, which begin to make available the courses and seminars of the years of gestation. It is particularly intriguing to see concrete evidence of Heidegger struggling with Husserl on the one hand and Aristotle on the other to find his own way.

This evolution has been studied in detail by Thomas Sheehan (1981, 1982). He has argued that the Being whose meaning Heidegger has sought is always that of beings (i.e., of "entities," of the things that are) and from the beginning was experienced as the disclosure of what is disclosed; that it was Husserl who helped Heidegger to see and formulate this; that this disclosure is eventually a disclosive process—a movement toward disclosure, profoundly "kinetic" in character; that it was Aristotle who helped him explore this kinetic quality through the notion of *kinēsis;* that in Heidegger's analysis of Aristotelian *kinēsis* one finds the essential elements of what he later called *Ereignis* or "event of appropriation."

For Aristotle, entities of nature (as opposed to artifacts made by man) are essentially in movement by reason of their very Being— their movement *is* their Being. This movement is a continued coming-into-presence that implies a whence and a whither of that coming, hence a relative absence (a "not-yet and a no-longer") intrinsic to the phenomenon. The double absencing intrinsic to the presencing process constitutes the movement, hence the Being of such entities. Sheehan calls it "pres-ab-sentiality" (1981, p. 537).

Heidegger finds this same structure in Aristotle's conception of *dynamis,* which does not mean for him abstract "possibility" but rather power-to-be (i.e., presence) that is imperfect (i.e., involves absence). The notion of *dynamis* rejoins the notion of *kinēsis,* then, and in a 1928 seminar Heidegger translated the former as *Eignung* and the latter as *Ereignung,* indicating how these two Greek words are ingredient to the word that would become central for him as his thought developed: *Ereignis.* What is at stake is a conception of Being as the process of disclosure that includes an absence intrinsic to its presencing. This absential component of the presencing process Heidegger expressed in many ways—for example, as *-lēthē* (-velation) interior to *a-lētheia* (re-velation), as *Verbergung* (concealment) interior to *Unverborgenheit* (revealment), as *Enteignis* (non-appropriation) interior to *Ereignis* (event of appropriation). In any case, this privative, absential component of the disclosive process within beings is ingredient to their

Being (for Heidegger, not just the Being of natural things but of all beings), and must be recognized if one is to respond to them appropriately.

Man's being, too, is characterized by the same kind of absential presencing, and it is by virtue of such a movement (of "transcendence") that he has access to other beings. Since the absential component of the movement that constitutes man's being may be considered in terms either of his coming-to-be (*Zukunft*) or of his having-beenness (*Gewesenheit*), the three ecstases of time (present, future, past) are reducible to the two components of movement: presencing and absencing. All of *Being and Time* is fundamentally an analysis of human being in these terms. And the famous "turn" in Heidegger's thinking, according to Sheehan, does not consist first of all in a shift of focus in Heidegger's thought during the thirties but rather of a "transformation of one's philosophical awareness into an effective recognition of the privative dimension of disclosure" (1981, p. 539), whether in human being itself or the other beings with which it deals. In *Being and Time*, the transformation goes by the name of "resolve," later by the name of "thought," or "release" (*Gelassenheit*), that is, a "letting oneself go along with the autodisclosure of entities" (1981, p. 540).

Be that as it may, the point to be made here is that Being thus experienced as the presencing-absencing disclosure of *Ereignis* is as de-substantified and de-ontified as one can conceive. The essential is that absence is ingredient to presence and that this pres-absenc-ing is temporal in structure. Let us return for a moment to the lecture of 1962. What was its theme? The old one: the relation of Being to Time. Heidegger's thesis: we cannot say that Being "is," nor that Time "is," for that would be to make them entities (*Seiende*). At best we must say: "Being is given," "Time is given." And what is it that does the giving? *Ereignis!* Note:

1. The giving includes the complementarity of presence and absence.

> We . . . find in absence—be it what has been or what is to come—a manner of presencing and approaching which by no means coincides with presencing in the sense of the imme-

diate present (*Gegenwart*). . . . Approaching, being not yet present, at the same time gives and brings about what is no longer present, the past, and conversely what has been offers future to itself. [1972, p. 13/14]

2. The giving implies reciprocity with the nature of man.

Man: standing within the approach of presence, but in such a fashion that he receives the coming-to-presence, the There-is-given, as gift, in the sense that he accepts what shines forth in letting-come-to-presence. If man were not the constant receiver of the gift by which "presence-is-given," if what is reached out to man in the gift did not reach him, then by default of this gift Being would not only be concealed, indeed it would not only be closed off, but man would be excluded from the entire reach of Being-is-given. Man would not be man. [1972, p. 12/12–13, slightly emended]

And as with Being, so with Time:

True time is the nearness of presencing out of present, having-been-ness and future that unifies the three-fold [mode of] luminous reaching forth. It has already so reached man as such that he can be man only insofar as he stands within the three-fold reaching and withstands the refusing-with-holding nearness that determines this reaching. [1972, p. 16/17, slightly emended]

3. Reduced to simplicity, then, the process, inasmuch as it involves the withholding of past and future from the present, comports negation, a withdrawal intrinsic to the event of appropriation (*Ereignis*) itself.

4. Finally, "this [event of appropriation] is not something new but the most ancient of the ancients in Western thought, the primal ancient that hides under the name *Alethēia*" (1969, p. 25, my translation).

We conclude, then, that the experience of *Ereignis* of the late years, with all the complexity of its formulation, retained the essentially kinetic, self-disclosive, self-retentive quality of Heidegger's reading of Aristotle's *kinēsis*. How is this helpful to psycho-analysis? I suggest that it permits us to think of the Other in the dimension of Being without hypostasizing it, or ontifying it, or absolutizing it in any way, first and foremost because it suggests a way to consider the unconscious as a disclosive process. If the unconscious "is" at all, it is a disclosure to man, as presence made up of absence, in such fashion that the withdrawal of *Ereignis* may be experienced as a form of negation, as No-thing (*Nichts*) without being absolutely nothing (hence, perhaps, as *béance?*)—subsisting in the "ex-sistence du dire." More specifically, there are at least three ways in which this conception might be suggestive.

In the first place, the conception of Being as *Ereignis-Alētheia* suggests a fresh way to meditate the essential nature of language. According to Heidegger, the pre-Socratics experienced the pres-abs-encing of Being, whether as *physis*, as *alētheia*, as *nomos*, and so forth, but never thematized it as such. That is why for Heraclitus "*physis* loves to hide itself." But the disclosive process is also *Logos*, and it was Heidegger's essay on *Logos* according to Heraclitus (Fragment B 50) that Lacan translated for his students in 1956.

As Heidegger reads Heraclitus, *Logos*, as noun, must be understood in terms of the verb form *legein*, as a laying down or out or side by side, hence a gathering into collectedness that lets what has thus been gathered together lie forth as what it is. If this be the process of the verb *legein*, what, then, is the *Logos*? It is the primal power from which the entire gathering process proceeds. Heidegger claims that Heraclitus' formula (*Hen-panta*: One-many), which occurs paratactically in the same fragment, describes the manner in which *Logos* functions. As the One (*Hen*), *Logos* is the gathering process that makes all beings (*panta*: the many) cohere within themselves and mesh with each other in an ordered pattern. *Logos* as the One is likened to a lightning bolt, by reason of which beings (the many) are lit up in their Being (1954, p. 72/222). What is the role of man in this process? His task is to collaborate in the gathering, to correspond with the *legein* of the *Logos* as *homologein*. I interpret this to mean that man is that being among the many others *where* the lightning bolt flashes forth to light up the rest of beings.

What has all this to do with language? Here Heidegger's thesis is radical and unequivocal: the sense of *legein*, which unquestionably means for the Greeks "to speak" and "to say," does not pass from one meaning (e.g., "letting-lie-forth-in-self-disclosure") to another (e.g., "to speak"), but the original sense of "speaking" is nothing less than "to let lie forth": "Saying and speaking occur essentially as [the process of] letting-lie-forth-in-collectedness everything that comes-to-presence [precisely inasmuch] as [it is] laid out in nonconcealment" (1954, p. 63/212). Thus, for Heidegger the essence of language is not to be sought first of all in terms of sound or meaning as these are dealt with either by linguists or language analysts but in the complete identification between bringing into words and letting-be-disclosed. We get a sense of what is meant when he explains the significance of "naming" something: "To name means to call forward. That which is gathered and laid down in the name, by means of such a laying, comes to light and comes to lie before us. The naming (*onoma*), thought in terms of *legein*, is not the expression of a word-meaning but rather a letting-lie-forth in the light where something stands in such a way that it has a name" (1954, p. 73/223).

Naming in this fashion is the special prerogative of poets, to be sure, but it is not restricted to them. We recall the familiar story of Helen Keller's first experience of the meaning of language: she had been taught to spell words like w-a-t-e-r in sign language that she could repeat in "monkey-like" fashion without knowing it was a word at all. One day, however,

> We walked down the path to the well-house, attracted by the fragrance of the honeysuckle with which it was covered. Someone was drawing water and my teacher placed my hand under the spout. As the cool stream gushed over one hand she spelled into the other the word w-a-t-e-r, first slowly and then rapidly. I stood still, my whole attention fixed upon the motions of her fingers. Suddenly I felt a misty consciousness as if something forgotten—a thrill of returning thoughts; and somehow the mystery of language was revealed to me. I knew then that "w-a-t-e-r" meant the wonderful cool some-

thing that was flowing over my hand. That living word awakened my soul, and gave it light, joy, set it free! [1922, p. 23]

Such, I argue, is what Heidegger would call the original and authentic function of language, to name beings in correspondence with the *Logos,* letting beings become manifest as what they are by letting them come into words.

Lacan acknowledges the power of naming. "As soon as [something] can be named, its presence can be evoked as an original dimension, distinct from reality. Nomination is an evocation of presence and maintains presence in absence" (1954–55, p. 297).

It is by nomination that man makes objects subsist with a certain consistency. . . . The [naming] word does not respond to the spatial distinction of the object . . . but to its temporal dimension. . . . [The] appearance [of the object] which [lasts] a certain time is recognizable, strictly speaking, only by the intermediary of the name. The name is the time of the object. [1954–55, p. 202]

For Lacan, naming in this fashion implies more than corresponding with the *Logos.* There is required, too, the functioning of the symbolic order—"It is there that the symbolic relation intervenes," for "naming constitutes a pact by which two subjects agree at the same time to recognize the same object" (1954–55, p. 202). What I am suggesting, then, is that if we are to read these texts in Heideggerian fashion, then the symbolic order would be first among the *panta* of Heraclitus which is disclosed *not by a metalanguage* but by *Logos* as *Hen.*

A second use for the Heideggerian notion of Being as *Ereignis-Alētheia* lies precisely in the withdrawing, self-concealing, absential aspect of the presencing of *Alētheia.* For Lacan has insisted much—along with Freud—on the inevitable distortions that are part of the psychoanalytic process: errors, mistakes, parapraxias, disguises, distortions, resistances, and so on, through which the unconscious recalcitrantly reveals itself (see 1953–54, p. 59). If "it is with the appearance of language that the dimension of truth emerges" (1977, p. 172/524), then with language—i.e., with the symbolic order—comes the lie, for "the man who in the act of speaking breaks the bread of truth with his counterpart also shares the lie" (1966, p. 379).

What kind of truth can this be that emerges shot through and through with un-truth? How does it emerge out of the ex-centric center of the subject if this center is the symbolic order only? What is the nature of the symbolic order if it yields a truth that comports its own negativity? Here again, Heidegger's conception of *Ereignis-Alētheia* can help.

There is no need to summarize here the discussion of truth in *Being and Time*. There truth as conformity between judgment and judged is shown to be grounded in the disclosive process of *Dasein,* that is, human being itself, where every apprehension (*Ergreifen*) is a mis-apprehension (*Vergreifen*), every dis-covery (*Entdecken*) a covering-over (*Verdecken*), every dis-closure (*Erschliessen*) a closing-over (*Verschliessen*) (1962a, p. 264/222, emended). We recall, too, the argument from the essay "On the Essence of Truth," where truth is meditated for itself, so to speak, rather than in terms of the finitude of *Dasein*. But it is impossible for Heidegger to meditate the essence of truth without at the same time considering the essence of un-truth. If truth as *Alētheia* is an unveiling, the veiling (*-lēthē*), too, must be questioned. It takes two forms: the concealing of the concealment (what Heidegger calls "mystery") and the confounding or compounding of this already concealed concealment in what he calls *die Irre* ("errancy").

Oblivious of the concealment of concealment (the mystery), *Dasein*'s ex-sistence becomes absorbed in the beings about it. The result is that *Dasein* wanders from one being to another in a state of confusion, driven about hither and thither, looking for the satisfaction that no being can give, searching for a repose that no being, torn from the roots of ultimate meaning and mystery, can offer. This is what is meant by "errancy." The condition of errancy is not occasional or accidental to *Dasein* but belongs to its "inner constitution" (1977a, pp. 135–36/196–97). The structural errancy of *Dasein* will be the ground of error to which *Dasein* falls prey.

"Error" in this case, however, means more than just a single mistake; it signifies the whole entangled complex of ways and means by which *Dasein* in its wandering can go astray. After all, every kind of comportment will have its own way of wandering about in forgetfulness of the mystery. The kingdom of error extends from such phenomena as a single mistake, oversight, or miscalculation up to the aberrations and excesses in matters of supreme moment. What one ordinarily calls "error," that is, the incorrectness of a judgment or falsity of knowledge, is only one way—for that matter, the most superficial way—in which *Dasein* goes astray. Furthermore, the errancy in which man walks is marked by a certain spontaneity of its own. "By leading him astray, errancy dominates man through and through" (1977a, p. 136/197).

Heidegger finds this negativity of truth even in Plato—for example, in the darkness of the cave after the prisoner returns. In this he claims that Plato remains faithful to the original experience of *Alētheia* of its predecessors (1962b). Again, later, when he meditates Heraclitus' notion of *polemos,* the primordial struggle out of which all things emerge, it is not just a conflict of opposites such as Jung experienced it to be, but the fundamental contention between concealment and revealment in *Alētheia* (1961, p. 51/47; 1977a, p. 180/49). Likewise, "*Logos* is *in itself* and *at the same time* a revealing and a concealing. . . . Unconcealment needs concealment, *Lēthē,* as a reservoir upon which disclosure can, as it were, draw" (1975, p. 71/221, Heidegger's italics). This concealment takes two forms: *Logos* withdraws in the beings it reveals, e.g., in the words that are just brought to expression. This means that there is a "not" in every word, behind which Being as *Logos* retreats. This constitutes the domain of the un-said, immanent in everything that is said (as Lacan finds to have been the case with Freud). We recognize here the essentials of Being-as-mystery. But the negativity of Being in language is such that it not only remains as such, withdrawing in words, but it even dupes man into disregarding it: "That is to say, [*Logos*] plays in such a way with our speaking process that it gladly lets our language wander astray in the more obvious meanings of words. It is as if man had difficulty in dwelling authentically in language" (1968, p. 118/83, emended).

When Lacan tells us that "error is the habitual incarnation of truth," and that "it would not be necessary to push things much farther to see here a constituting structure of the revelation of Being as such" (1953–54, pp. 289–90), how can that be explained by the pluses and minuses, the zeros and ones, the yeses and nos of the *jeu combinatoire*? I am suggesting instead that the conception of *Ereignis-Alētheia* offers us a way to make sense out of how "the internal necessity of error" (1953–54, p. 291) is ingredient to the "constituting structure of the revelation of Being as such."

The third value for psychoanalysis in the conception of Being as *Ereignis-Alētheia* may be seen in Heidegger's reading of Parmenides and has to do with the nature of desire. We recall how Lacan conceives the role of desire in psychoanalysis. For him, "the world of Freud is not the world of things, nor the world of Being but the world of desire as such" (1954–55, p. 261). What the *cogito* was for Descartes, the *desidero* is for Freud. "It is from there, necessarily, that the essential of primary process is constituted" (1964, p. 154/141). Desire in the properly human sense begins only with the infant's separation from the purely dual relationship with its mother at the time that it begins to speak. Perhaps the quickest way to get a grasp on what Lacan means by desire is to return to that moment of the *fort-da* experience when the child, with its game of disappearance and return, renders present what is absent (the mother) through the phonemes of inchoate speech. Lacan tells us that the moment when the child is "born into language" is likewise that in which "desire becomes human" (1977, p. 103/319). What does it mean for "desire to become human" at that time? Lacan leaves us to our own resources here, but I take him to mean that up to that time the child seeks only the satisfaction of bodily needs and to that extent is hardly different from any animal organism. For him this is not desire, but only "need." Desire emerges as a specifically human phenomenon with the infant's birth into language because it is at that point that he first experiences "want." Up to that time the infant has been engaged with the mother in an essentially *dual*

relationship—a quasi-symbiotic tie that prolongs psychologically
the physical symbiosis in the womb. But with the *fort-da* experience, that tie is ruptured, and the child experiences the trauma of
limitation—or as Lacan puts it, a *manque à être*.

The word *manque* here is polyvalent. In French, *manque* may
mean "lack," "deficiency," or "want." Hence, *manque à être* would
mean "lack of being," or "deficiency in regard to being," or the
state of being "in want of being." But this "being in want of" being
may be understood also as "wanting" being, so that the most
recent English translator—at Lacan's own bidding (1977, p. ix)—
renders *manque à être* as "want to be." It is precisely this "want to
be" that I take to be the sense of what Lacan means by "desire." As
to the nature of the "being" of which the child is in want once the
purely imaginary sense of completeness through union with the
mother has been ruptured, Lacan tells us nothing, though the
problem will return under the guise of what he eventually calls
the *objet a*.

Torn from a dyadic relationship with its mother, the infant
must now relate to her through what Lacan calls a "dialectic of
desire," in which the subject's ultimate quest is for recognition by
the desired. Here, the phrase "dialectic of desire" suggests Hegel
more than Heidegger, and we recall how for Hegel the dialectical
movement by which the individual "I" becomes self-conscious
proceeds through a dynamism of desire, the central theme of
which is that what the "I" desires is to be the desire of the other
whom he desires—to be desired in turn, to be recognized as desir-
able by the other. "The desire of man is the desire of the Other"
(1953–54, p. 169), as we are told again and again.

In any case, traumatized by its want, the child wants—desires—
to recapture its lost paradise by being the desired of its mother,
her fullness—in Lacanian language, by being the phallus for its
mother. Alas, that is impossible, for the father is there: the real
father, the imaginary father, and most of all the symbolic father—the "law of the father," the symbolic order structuring all
human relationships, including now the relationship with its
mother. Henceforth, the child's desire must be articulated
through the metonymic linkage of the signifiers that constitute its

symbolic chain, "like rings in a necklace that is the ring in another necklace made of rings."

Now the interpretation of desire as desire of the Other in Hegelian fashion is successful as far as it goes and certainly finds clinical confirmation, particularly when one takes as its paradigm, as Lacan does, the dialectic of master and slave. But can one take part of Hegel without taking all of him? Clearly, Lacan later refuses to go the full way with Hegel to the point of accepting successive syntheses in a movement toward Absolute Knowledge (e.g., 1964, p. 221/201). In any case, I propose here a Heideggerian reading of the "desire of the Other," partly for its complementary value, in order to sound the full Heideggerian overtones of the whole.

In the *Introduction to Metaphysics* Heidegger meditates Parmenides' gnome (Fragment 5), *to gar auto noein estin te kai einai* in terms of the relation between Being (*einai*) and man (*noein*) as one (*auto*)—that is, as mutually correlative. Later, in *What Is Called Thinking?*, he returns to the same theme in another text of Parmenides (Fragment 6), *chrē: to legein te noein t': emmenai* (1968, p. 175 and passim), and translates the Greek *chrē* (often grossly rendered by "it is necessary") by *es brauchet*—"there is want of." In other words, being is "in want of" man's *legein-noein* (thought). Later, Heidegger interpreted *Moira* in Parmenides as the apportionment (*Zuteilung*) to man that proceeds from this want (1975, p. 97/251). "Want" here echoes what in the *Introduction to Metaphysics* was called Being's "need" (*Not*) for *Dasein* (e.g., 1961, pp. 136–37, 148, and passim). Man responds to this want by a want (*Mögen*) of his own by reason of which he is empowered to respond to Being's want through thought: "Only when we want [*mögen*] what in itself is most to-be-thought are we empowered [*vermögen*] to think" (1968, p. 4/1, emended).

This correlation between Being's want and the empowering of *Dasein* is even more explicit in the "Letter on Humanism." Here the want of being is expressed by *mögen* (normally: to be willing, to desire or have a mind to, to like, etc.). The English translator renders it by "favor"—legitimate choice, no doubt, but lacking the force of *chrē: es brauchet*. At the risk of some violence, I prefer to use "want" for *mögen* in the text in question.

The context of the letter is clear. Jean Beaufret has asked if for Heidegger a humanism is still possible, and Heidegger responds by articulating his conception of man as essentially open to being. We recall how in *Being and Time* this had been analyzed as *Dasein's Möglichkeit*, or *Seinsvermögen*, i.e., *Dasein's dynamis* or *kinēsis*, his power-(drive-)to-be. The passage in question reads:

> Being has taken [*annehmen*] thought in its essence [i.e., *Dasein*] unto itself. . . . But to take a "thing" or a "person" in its essence unto oneself may mean to "love" [*lieben*] or "want" [*mögen*] it. Thought in a more original way, such wanting means to bestow essence as a gift [*das Wesen schenken*]. Such wanting is the genuine essence of empowering [*Vermögens*] something to be. . . . It is on the "strength" of this wanting-that-empowers [*Vermögen des Mögens*] that something is genuinely empowered to be. . . . Out of this wanting, Being empowers thought [*Dasein*]. [1977a, p. 196/148, slightly emended]

What I take Heidegger to be saying here is that it is because Being first wants (*mögen*) *Dasein* that it empowers *Dasein* (*vermögen*) as power-to-be (*Seinsvermögen*), which in its structural unity is designated in *Being and Time* as "care" (*Sorge*) for the Being of beings.

In other words, it is through *Dasein* that being adheres to itself and it is this adherence of Being to Being through *Dasein* that I take to be the dynamic of *Dasein's* desire. Obviously this desire is filtered through other *Daseins*. Dasein never ek-sists alone but is always with other *Daseins* in the world. Essentially (so I interpret Heidegger in paraphrasing a classic formula), "the desire with which *Desein* desires Being is the desire by which Being desires *Dasein*." When we hear Lacan say, then, that the desire of man is the desire of the Other, where Other is capitalized and taken to mean the unconscious, I am suggesting that we hear that in Heideggerian fashion as saying that desire is "of" the Other in the double sense of both an objective and subjective genetive: desire is of the Other in the sense that it is both for the Other and from the Other, coursing through man as his *dynamis* with a different center than his I-saying Cartesian subjectivity.

Is this really helpful? It certainly seems necessary for Lacan if

he wants a "dialectic of desire" (broad sense) without the "successive syntheses" that a thoroughly consequent Hegelianism would
impose. Second, it is necessary for the thesis that I am venturing
here—namely, that the Other as Lacan conceives it must be explored philosophically, at least in a first moment of reflection, in
terms of Heidegger's experience of being as *Ereignis-Alētheia*. For
Freud's world is a world of desire, and no philosophical reflection
would be adequate that did not take account of this dimension.
The conception of desire that a Heideggerian reading makes
possible is that of a dynamism (transcendence) that is ineluctably
finite, scarred by a double absence—a past that it is-as-having-
been and an indefinite future that comes to it in incessant withdrawal into beings that always disappoint and are strung together
metonymically like rings of a necklace that is a ring in another
necklace made of rings.

Finally, this conception may eventually be of some technical
service when the time comes to orchestrate more fully the meaning of the relationship between the subject and the Other that
Lacan describes in terms of "alienation"/"separation." His own
formulations utilize such concepts as "union" (or "joining") and
"intersection" (1978, p. 213/194), drawn from the theory of sets.
If it is possible to think this problem according to a philosophical
rather than a mathematical paradigm, one may wonder if the
right place to start may not be the notion of *Moira* in Parmenides—that is, with what Heidegger translates as *Zuteilung* (apportionment) and understands as the "destining" (*Geschick*) of being,
where Being is in want of man who, by this very fact, is empowered to want (desire) Being in return, because of the correlative finitude of both.

Is all this a futile effort, doomed to sterility, inasmuch as by his
own subsequent acknowledgment Lacan's use of Heidegger's
thought was no more than a "propaedeutic reference"? I suggest
that it is more than that. Lacan's voice now is silent, and his oral
teaching has passed into the written word—a corpus of his *énoncés*. If his work is to be more than a deposit of faith to be
elaborated by a pious scholasticism into a system of Absolute
Knowledge, then the task is not simply to explicate further his

énoncés, but to try to return to the moment of *énonciation* when the speaking subject called Jacques Lacan was at his very best. But this means trying to articulate his un-said, learning to read him as he has taught us to read Freud, finding as he did in Freud's un-said the intuitions of structural linguistics. This type of re-trieve (*Wiederholung*) is fraught with peril, of course, but all true thought is a risk—and Heidegger is a good mentor.

Furthermore, this kind of effort, however tentative, is worth making for the sake of psychoanalysis itself. For it would seem that psychoanalysis cannot make a complete rupture with philosophy except at cost to itself. I speak of "philosophy," not "metaphysics," meaning by that that the Being-question must eventually be posed for psychoanalysis at least to the extent of illuminating its "imperceptible, inaccessible, ineluctable" ground (1977b). What I have suggested here is that the Being of the symbolic order is not an ontic Other of the Other like a Super-Absolute, but the disclosure of the Other as such in *kinēsis*—in *Ereignis-Alētheia*—which, as *Logos*, is aboriginal language. This implies both revealment and concealment. To the extent that the moment of revealment can be frozen into an ontic present in the thematizing of scientific abstraction, the analysis of the Other in terms of language could indeed yield the synchronic structure that linguists discern. But to the extent that it remains a *kinēsis*, marked by a double absence, it would make diachrony or history possible—not simply the individual history of the particular subject but Being-as-history (*Seinsgeschichte*) as such, and this would enable us to think of how there may be a special place in it for someone like Jacques Lacan. He seemed, and had a right, to expect that place.

REFERENCES

De Waelhens, A. *La philosophie de Martin Heidegger*. Louvain: Institut Supèrieur de Philosophie, 1942.
Freud, S. *Beyond the Pleasure Principle* (1920). *Standard Edition of the Complete Psychological Works*, vol. 18. London: Hogarth, 1955.

Heidegger, M.
  Introduction to Metaphysics. Translated by R. Manheim. Garden City,
    N.Y.: Doubleday (Anchor), 1961. (*Einführung in die Metaphysik.*
    Tübingen: Niemyer, 1953.)
  Being and Time (1927). Translated by J. Macquarrie and E. Robinson.
    New York: Harper & Row, 1962a. (*Sein und Zeit.* Frankfurt:
    Niemeyer, 1977.)
  "Plato's Doctrine of Truth." Translated by J. Barlow. In *Philosophy in
    the Twentieth Century,* vol. 3. Edited by W. Barrett and H. D. Aiken.
    New York: Random House, 1962b. ("Platons Lehre von der
    Wahrheit." In *Wegmarken.* Frankfurt: Klostermann, 1976.)
  What Is Called Thinking? Translated by F. D. Wieck and J. G. Gray. New
    York: Harper & Row, 1968. (*Was Heisst Denken?* Tübingen:
    Niemeyer, 1954.)
  On Time and Being. Translated by J. Stambaugh. New York: Harper &
    Row, 1972. ("Zeit und Sein." In *Zur Sache des Denkens.* Tübingen:
    Niemeyer, 1969.)
  "Preface" to W. J. Richardson (1974).
  "Logos" (Heraclitus Fragment B 50). Translated by D. F. Krell.
    "Moira" (Parmenides VIII, 34–41). Translated by F. A. Capuzzi.
    Both in *Early Greek Thinking.* New York: Harper & Row, 1975. (Both
    in *Vorträge und Aufsätze.* Pfullingen: Neske, 1954.)
  "On the Essence of Truth." Translated by J. Sallis. "The Origin of the
    Work of Art." Translated by A. Hofstadter. "Letter on Humanism."
    Translated by F. A. Capuzzi. All three in *Basic Writings.* Edited by D.
    F. Krell. New York: Harper & Row, 1977a. ("Vom Wesen der
    Wahrheit" and "Brief über den Humanismus." In *Wegmarken.*
    Frankfurt: Klostermann, 1976.) ("Der Ursprung des Kunstwerkes."
    In *Holzwege.* Frankfurt: Klostermann, 1977.)
  "Science and Reflection." Translated by W. Lovitt. In *The Question
    Concerning Technology: Heidegger's Critique of the Modern Age.* New
    York: Harper & Row, 1977b. ("Wissenschaft und Besinnung." In
    Vorträge und Aufsätze. Pfullingen: Neske, 1954.)
Keller, H. *The Story of My Life.* New York: Doubleday, Page, 1922.
Lacan, J.
  Le Séminaire: Livre I. Les Écrits Techniques de Freud (1953–54). Paris:
    Seuil, 1975.
  *Le Séminaire: Livre II. Le moi dans la théorie de Freud et dans la technique de
    la psychanalyse* (1954–55). Paris: Seuil, 1978.

Translation of "Logos," by M. Heidegger. *La Psychanalyse* 1 (1956): 59–79.

The Four Fundamental Concepts of Psycho-Analysis (1964). Translated by A. Sheridan. New York: Norton, 1978.

Le Séminaire: Livre XX. Encore (1972–73). Paris: Seuil, 1975.

Écrits: A Selection. Translated by A. Sheridan. New York: Norton, 1977. (*Écrits.* Paris: Seuil, 1966.)

Richardson, W. J. *Heidegger: Through Phenomenology to Thought.* 3d ed. The Hague: Nijhoff, 1974.

Sheehan, T. "On Movement and the Destruction of Ontology." *The Monist* 64 (1981): 534–42.

———. "Heidegger's Philosophy of Mind." In *Chroniques de la Philosophie.* Edited by P. Ricoeur. 1982, in preparation.

8

Logic of Lacan's *objet (a)** and Freudian Theory: Convergences and Questions

ANDRÉ GREEN

Since Lacan's work is beginning to spread over the English-speaking world, and provokes some curiosity, an essay bearing witness to the kind of discussions which took place in the frame of his seminar during the sixties may be of interest, even though its author has not been a follower of the Lacanian movement for more than a decade. Apart from the style, obviously influenced by Lacan's deliberately elliptic and poetic way of exposition, the content of this chapter may provoke resistance and rejection— not only because of basic disagreements, but also because the concepts used here (psychoanalytical and nonpsychoanalytical) are usually foreign to Anglo-Saxon psychoanalytic tradition. However, a short foreword may facilitate its reading by providing information on the circumstances of its birth and the context in which it was presented for the first time.

When I started my psychoanalytical training in 1955 I had chosen the Société Psychanalytique de Paris, which Lacan had left during the first split in 1953. I had met Lacan personally on different occasions but was hesitant to attend his public seminar at Sainte-Anne's Hospital, where I used to work. It was not until

Translated by Kimberly Kleinart and Beryl Schlossman. This essay is an expanded version of a lecture given in a seminar of Jacques Lacan's, 21 December 1965. It was first published in *Cahiers pour l'Analyse*, 1966 (3) (Seuil). Reprinted by permission.

Editors' note: Green's use of "*objet(a)*" is further discussed in Kerrigan's introduction to this volume.

1960, after my participation in the meeting organized in Bonneral by Henri Ey—the most famous and justly celebrated French psychiatrist—on the Unconscious that I decided to attend Lacan's seminar. In Bonneral the first public confrontation took place in which Lacan and his followers (mainly Laplanche and Leclaire) faced members of the Société Psychanalytique de Paris, of which I was a young member. In my discussion of Laplanche and Leclaire's important contribution, based on Lacan's ideas, I emphasized the absence of any reference to affect in their structural view. This point is brought out again in the following pages.

Convinced of the importance of Lacan's teachings, I decided to attend his seminar in the fall of 1960. In 1964, after the second split, which led to the dissolution of the Société Française de Psychanalyse and the creation of the Association Psychanalytique de France (Lagache, Laplanche, and others), affiliated to the International Psychoanalytical Association and the Ecole Freudienne in Paris founded by Jacques Lacan, Lacan's seminar moved to the Ecole Normale Superieure. Hence his public now included many young philosophers (students of the Ecole Normale Superieure), who were intrigued and attracted by this unusual presentation of the psychoanalytic concepts to which until then they had paid little attention because of their philosophical inconsistency. Lacan decided that some sessions of his seminar, which was open to the public, would thenceforward be restricted to discussions in a smaller group. He invited those who wished to discuss the contents of his seminar to present their remarks or their objections. It was during one of these "closed seminars" that the following work was presented, at Lacan's request. My contribution was a critical one, but as it was a psychoanalytic discussion, not a philosophical one, it differed from the others. Those of the audience who were psychoanalysts were in large majority disciples of Lacan. The few analysts who were not among his followers kept silent. But all shared an interest in trying to think of the concepts of psychoanalysis in terms of their philosophical implications.

At the time, Lacan's stimulating work compelled those who were interested in his views to be familiar with the main currents of the movement of ideas in the sixties, such as Saussure's work in linguistics, Lévi-Strauss's in anthropology, and so forth. This explains the reference to their work, inasmuch as all of them, explicitly or implicitly, made use of a conception of the unconscious which was quite different, it seemed to me, from the psychoanalytic one.

One can hardly imagine how alive, how passionate these discussions were. At the time, Lacan's seminars were unpublished, so everyone had to rely on the faithfulness of his memory or on some scanty notes. That explains why the review in the first part of the paper was a necessary step. Lacan's *Écrits,* his collected papers, were not issued until 1966, after the presentation of my work. I would like to add that the approximation of our understanding and the moderate reliability of our memory was largely compensated by an extraordinary enthusiasm and a high level of attention.

In 1967 my participation in Lacan's seminar stopped, for reasons I cannot explain here. The great sophistication of Lacan's theory could no longer mask for me the fact that many clinical and technical problems were ignored or left out by the master. Further, I was already paying great attention to the works of Winnicott and Bion. Their richness was not limited to brilliant rhetoric, and it was directly in touch with clinical experience and the new problems that psychoanalysts have to face with the changes in psychoanalytic practice.

Nevertheless, I regard those years 1960–67 as an important step in my training, even though I had to come to the conclusion that Lacan's way was not mine.

In discussion of the object of psychoanalysis, one question immediately comes to mind: Will we consider the object of psychoanalysis as the object of a science (the focus of that science throughout its development), or will we talk about the object in terms of its psychoanalytical status? It would be somewhat surprising to show that these two meanings are closely related and even interdependent.

Littré calls our attention to the Academy's comment on the word *subject*: natural bodies constitute the subject of physics.

Again, under the word *object,* the Academy is quoted as saying that natural bodies are the object of physics. It is not my purpose here to point out a repetition that seems contradictory or that could be too easily dismissed. Nor will I conclude by lending my voice to the mass accusations of those who see the separation of subject and object as being the cause of all theoretical impasses for which traditional thought is deemed responsible.

To confront at the outset the related destinies of subject and object implies neither blending them together nor dissociating them for each other. It does imply that we will have to look closely at oppositions between identity and difference, between conjunction and disjunction, between suture and separation (*coupure*). We will then have to raise the question of whether or not the object of psychoanalysis (i.e., its end, or goal) can be satisfied with the limitations inherent in this structure of binary opposition—as so many of the more sophisticated contemporary disciplines seem to be.

Jacques Lacan's Object: An Overview

If we examine the role of the *objet (a)* in the theory of Jacques Lacan, we shall kill two birds with one stone. This will allow us, first, to delineate the content of the *objet (a)* within its own conceptual framework, and second, to mark out the limitations of the modern structuralist dimension of Lacanian thought and, no doubt, of all psychoanalytic thought.

THE OTHER (*le (a)*), MEDIATION BETWEEN THE SUBJECT AND THE OTHER (*l'Autre*)

The (*a*) (I will specify the *objet (a)* at a later point) is present in Lacan's earliest graph (see figure, Schéma L),[1] in which he takes as his starting point the theorization given in the *Stade du miroir* (1936–49). (*a*), in its relation to *a'* (which will be closely related to the future i(*a*), i.e., the mirror image), can be understood as an *element of ineluctable mediation* uniting the subject with the Other.

---

1. This graph, Schéma L, is reproduced in the introduction to "Seminaire sur la lettre volée," *La Psychanalyse,* vol. 2, p. 9.

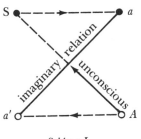

Schéma L

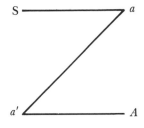

Schéma L simplified

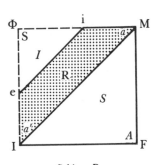

Schéma R

A: the Other
I: the Imaginary
I: ego ideal
M: signifier of the primordial object (mother)
F: position of the *Name-of-the-Father* in the locus of the Other
S: Subject
S: the Symbolic
R: the Real
Φ: phallus (Imaginary object)

i ⎫ the two Imaginary endpoints of all later narcissistic relationships, the ego
e ⎭ (e) and the specular image (i)

segment iM (on the line SM, Si, Sa^1, Sa^2, Sa^3, . . . SM): the axis of
    desires (object choice)

a: Objects—figure of the Imaginary other of the mirror stage segment eI (on the
    line SI, Se, Sa^1, Sa^2, Sa^3, . . . SI): the axis of identification (narcissism)

a': the identification of the (child's) ego through the identification with the ideal
    of the ego (the paternal imago), i.e., identification of the ego on the path of
    the paternal identification with the ego ideal

EDITORS' NOTE: See also Lacan, 1977, pp. 193, 197; Wilden, 1968, pp. 107, 294;
Muller and Richardson, 1979, p. 391.

Clearly, the situation of the mirror stage (*le stade du miroir*)—
which it is less important to pinpoint chronologically as a stage
than to designate as a structuring situation—is only understandable if we note that it is psychoanalysis, not psychology, which is at
stake. It is psychoanalysis which gives to the child, woman born, a
significance bearing on his entire development: namely, that he is
the substitute for the penis of which the mother is deprived, and
that he can only achieve his status as subject by situating himself at
the point where he is missing from the mother on whom he
depends. This substitute is the location and link of exchange
between the mother and the father, who, possessing the penis,
still cannot create it (since he *has* it).

The relationship of (*a*) to i(*a*) will repeat the relationship I have
just described.

THE (*a*), MEDIATION FROM THE SUBJECT TO THE EGO IDEAL

Next comes the quadrangle called Schéma R.[2] Once again the
system of desires (iM) is opposed to the system of identifications
(eI). The (*a*) is inscribed on the line (iM) going from the subject S
toward the primordial object M (the Mother), and it takes shape
through the figures of the imaginary other. However, the *a'* is
inscribed on the line going from the subject to the ego ideal
through the mirror shapes of the ego. We see how the quadrangle
originates in the Z, whose points it connects—in the first graph
these points are reached only by an indirect route. I could point
out that in the zone of the imaginary, the subject goes in one of
two directions: either toward the object or toward the ideal. We
know that in Freudian thought this orientation is heavily dependent on narcissism. We may then make the following remark
about the Other: located at the *Name-of-the-Father*, entirely situated in the Symbolic field, at the pole opposite the subject (who is
identified with the phallus), the Other can be reached only by the
two paths just described, via the object or via narcissism. There is
no direct route to the Other.

2. This graph is introduced in "D'une question préliminaire à tout traitement
possible d'une psychose," *La Psychanalyse*, vol. 2, p. 22. ("On a Question Preliminary to Any Possible Treatment of Psychosis" [1955–56], in Lacan, 1977.)

The field of the real is included in the tension between the two couples eI × iM, the significance of which I have explained. But it is only in the field of the symbolic that the third term—crucial in the structuring of this process—appears.[3]

THE (*a*), OBJECT OF DESIRE

Actually, Lacan postulates the existence of an ideal ego as a precocious form of the identification of the self with certain objects which act simultaneously as love objects and as objects of identification, but insofar as they are uprooted, cut up, and set apart from a series which shows what's missing. I who speak, I identify you with the object which you yourself lack, says Lacan. The relationship between (*a*) and *A* is thereby more clearly demonstrated. If *A*, to attain its full significance, requires the support of the *Name-of-the-Father* (which is neither a name nor a God), it passes along the maternal route and becomes effective only when the break between the subject and the maternal object separates irremediably the two entities. Or, once again, when the lack, the "missing-ness," which affects the primordial object, reveals itself in the experience of castration. The series of castrations postulated by Freud—weaning, sphincter control, castration as such—gives this experience its signifying power (because of its repetition) as well as its structuring power (due to its recurrence). Thus, the *objet (a)* seems to detach itself from this series of experiences, as Lacan says, thereby falling from its position as "exhibitor in the field of the Other"[4] so that it attains the status of the object of desire. The price paid for this access is the exclusion of the desir-

3. Two comments may be useful at this point: (1) French psychoanalytical works (cf. the work of Bouvet) develop the notion of object relations, taken from Anglo-Saxon writings (the work of Melanie Klein especially, following the work of Abraham). Lacan refutes their perspective by pointing out the absence of any reference to elements of mediation in these conceptions. Above all, he condemns this view insofar as it leads to the opposition Real-Imaginary, by dismissing the Symbolic. (2) The opposition ideal ego vs. ego ideal (Nunberg-Lagache) serves as a basis for putting Lacan's theoretical developments into the perspective of the relation to the Other.

4. "Remarques sur le rapport de D. Lagache," *La Psychanalyse*, vol. 6, p. 145.

ing subject, making it possible to speak—to name—the object of desire.

The location of this object in the field of the Other allows us, therefore, to conceive of the function of mediation that such an object plays out, not so much *between* the subject and the Other, as in their relationship; my desire enters the Other who has awaited it, forever under the form of the object that I am—inasmuch as the Other exiles me from my subjectivity by including all signifiers—i.e., that to which this subjectivity is attached.[5]

We know that fantasy allows this structure of relationship to be established, insofar as that fantasy reveals the subject of this relationship even as it erases its tracks. Fantasy is thus the structure that constitutes the subject—on which the subject imprints itself negatively, and on which fascination operates, opening out the relationship of the *objet (a)* with the ideal ego.

THE FETISH (*a*)

This formulation indicates everything that distinguishes Lacan's theorization from that of other authors. Whereas they tend to stress the positive aspect of the characteristics of the object, Lacan emphasizes the negative approach. One clear-cut example demonstrates this. As regards the image of the phallic mother, post-Freudian authors say that she is terrifying *because* she is phallic. Since the phallus can be an instrument of evildoing, a destructive weapon, and so forth, Freud remarked that the stultifying effect (*sidération*) produced by the Medusa's head resulted from the fact that the reptiles taking the place of her hair *were denying castration as many times as there were snakes*. In this reversal, the subject engaged in annulling castration was reminded many times over of its reality. Lacan would tend to go along with the latter interpretation. The fable of this reflexive mode is the case of fetishism, which he explores at length. The fetish object is the witness, the veil—of the castrated genitals—of what is missing in the field of the Other.

---

5. Seminar on "L'Angoisse" (1963), unpublished.

THE (*a*), OBJECT OF WHAT IS MISSING, CAUSE OF DESIRE

The metonymic and metaphoric structure of the *objet (a)* comes across with particular emphasis in Lacan's seminar on the *Symposium*.[6] In his reading of Plato's text, Lacan singles out the particular position of the *agalmata* in Alcibiades' speech depicting Socrates: "He is just like the sileni one sees standing in sculpture workshops and which the artists depict holding a reed or a flute; were one to open them up from the middle, one would see that they contain figurines of the gods inside them." We are confronted simultaneously by the bodily fragment, by the body part and by its symbolization—and this is to be taken literally, in the form of the divine figurine.

It is precisely to the extent that this *objet (a)* comes forth as the object of lack (the *missing* object) that it will operate on two levels: as the revelation of the lack of the Other and as the lack appearing within the signifying process. That which is missing in the Other is that which one cannot conceive of. The $(-\Phi)$ which enters here in the guise of that which does not appear—that is, the Nothing which it is impossible to represent—organizes the confrontation with castration as that which is unthinkable: this gap in the possibilities of thought is filled in by the process of significance ("*significantisation*"), by the mirage of knowledge. Another quotation: "(*a*) symbolizes that which, in the realm of the signifier as lost, loses itself to "*significantisation*." It is the designated subject who resists this loss; at the moment the process of knowledge comes into play, at the moment of *knowing*, something is lost." This appearance in the form of the object of lack brings out the specific focus of our exposé, that is, *the nonspecularizable nature of the (a)*. The course of events is such that the barred subject takes on the function of i(*a*), according to Lacan's expression; or as if the subject short-circuiting the impossible specularization of lack were to identify itself with the knowledge which, emerging at the site of that loss which brings it into play, covers over this loss to the point of forgetting its existence.

6. Seminar on the *Symposium* (1960), unpublished.

Beginning with this appearance of lack, the function of the residue (*le reste*) stemming from the desire of the other—the residue which presents itself as the residue that has slipped past the bar—affects the great Other: the counterpart of this *reste* in the subject interests it in knowledge. There again Lacan makes a logical distinction, whereby nullification does not suppress the fact of possession (*l'avoir*), which brings about the appearance of the residue.

The function of the residue is saved from the threat hanging over the subject: "Desire is constructed in the pathway of a question: not to be, or the undoing of one's being born (*n'être*)." The *objet (a)* is the cause of desire.

(*a*), PRODUCT OF WORK

Although Lacan does not actually come out and say it, one might think that the progression-regression dimension constitutes an opposition related to those of conjunction-disjunction and the suture-cut. The developments as regards knowledge must be considered in their negative perspective, as referring to *méconnaissance* (a failure to know, or a misunderstanding), which organizes them in the process of *significantisation*—which tends to annul or nullify the loss of the object—and referring to that which is signified about this loss, given the traces of this work. The *objet (a)* will be the surest guideline, the indicator of truth pointing toward the subject. In his final writings, Freud stresses the *historical truth* upon which the analyst's "construction" focuses. The channel of asking (*la demande*) constitutes Ariadne's thread giving us access to truth. Its function is not only to serve as guideline, but also to map out this itinerary for the paths leading to truth.

This summary, reduced to the bare minimum necessary for understanding the developments which will follow, allows us to ask a few questions.

1. Given the relation of the *objet (a)* to *representation,* it is appropriate to investigate its relation to the signifying chain. What relationship is there between represented lack and speech as concatenation?
2. Must we follow Freud in assessing the status of the signifier only in terms of *Vorstellung-repräsentanz?* What about *affect?*

3. Is there not in Freud's work one point about representation which has not been taken up by Lacan: the distinction between *different types of representation* (e.g., that of words and of things), which might lead to still further differentiation, in order to underline the original character of Freudian concatenation?

4. If knowledge is that which comes forth in the place of truth, after loss of the object, shouldn't they be linked to one another by *the marks (traces) of this loss and the attempt to efface them*?

These questions will allow us to consider the *objet (a)* less as a support for the partial object than as the passage of a tracing hand: inscription, letter, *a*.

The Suture of the Signifier, Its Representation and the Objet (a)

We are approaching what will constitute another axis of my exposition—that is, the relationship linking (*a*) to cut and to suture. I will refer to the exposition by Jacques Alain Miller concerning the theorization of the logic of the signifier, starting with Frege's work;[7] I shall do so in order to specify the position of the number zero—that is, its pertinence regarding the fate of the (*a*).

By virtue of the principle that (in order to keep truth unthreatened) each thing is identical to itself and zero is the number assigned to the concept of "not identical to itself," no object corresponds to this concept.

But, objects Miller, in reference to Frege,

> In order to exclude any reference to the real, it was necessary to evoke, on a conceptual level, an object non-identical to itself—and then to evacuate it from the dimension of truth. The o inscribed at the site of the number consummates the exclusion of this object. At this site, demarcated by the subsuming which takes place, the object is lacking: nothing can be written here, and if one must mark an o, it is only as figuration of a blank spot, thereby rendering lack visible.

We have here on the one hand the evocation and the exclusion of the object non-identical to itself, and on the other, this blank spot, this hole, at the site of the subsumed object.

7. "La Suture," in *Cahiers pour l'Analyse*, no. 1.

The notion of unity is given by the concept of identity, the concept of the subsumed object. But its place as one, no longer as a unity but as number 1, remains problematic with respect to its place as first, or given what one might call its primordial quality.

Miller remarks that it is illegitimate to count the number zero as nothing, and logic would have us assign to this number zero the role of *first object*.

Consequently, the identification with the concept of the number zero subsumes the object number zero insofar as it is *one* object.* Thus, primordiality cannot be established under the aegis of unity, but only under that of the *number* which makes the 1 possible—the number zero. Thus, two levels of meaning recover an operation which must itself be articulated in order that we understand the ambiguity of the number zero, as regards its inclusion of:

• the concept of being non-identical to itself
• the object (matrix of the one) allowing the number 1 to be assigned.

The double operation is then uncovered:

• the evocation and eliding of the non-identical to itself, with a blank space at the level of the subsumed object permitting the number zero
• the introduction of the zero as a number, i.e., as a signifying name and as an object.

This situation is of interest in that it captures *the structure of concatenation.* Not only does the subject cut himself off from the signifying stage and from the signifying chain by the very fact of establishing it as a subject, within the structure of concatenation, but, furthermore, *the first of these objects* functions simultaneously as a concept and as an object, not represented but named as single object and as concept of non-identity to itself, *a concept that threatens truth,* insofar as it is not subject to questioning (*hors-jeu*) or not subjective (*hors-je*).

This truth-threatening concept is for us a concept resulting

---

*_Translators' note:_ A play here on the French *un* as meaning both "an" and "one" is lost in translation.

from *the meeting with truth,* in that it not only dissociates the truth from its demonstration (identity with itself) but it also indicates its place within truth as the blank space or the markings (*trace*) that negate it. It is inadequate to see this concept only as a simple relation to absence. The relationship *of lack to truth* must be specified.

What is at stake, for us, in the confrontation with Miller's reading of Frege is the tie between subject and signifier. The subject identifies with the repetition presiding over each of the operations through which concatenation knots itself, each fragment appropriated by the fragment preceding it and the one following it; at the same time and with the same gesture, the subject sees himself repeatedly ejected outside the scene—and the chain— which thereby constitutes itself. However, although the operation excludes this subject, *the act of nullification does not destroy the gain which seems to us to persist,* as long as we are able to recognize it in the form of the (*a*).

The effect of concatenation fits in with Lacan's definition of the signifier: "The signifier is that which represents a subject for another signifier." The relations between subject and *objet (a),* as regards suture and cut (or separation: *coupure*), are thereby clarified. "If in the series of numbers zero's metonymy begins with its metaphor," writes Miller, "if the number o of the series as number is only the suturing replacement of the absence (of absolute zero) which moves below the chain, following the alternating movement of a representation and of an exclusion, then what prevents us from recognizing, in the restored relationship of zero to the numeric series, the most basic articulation of the relationship that the subject maintains with the signifying chain?"

At this point I will not go into the zero's effect on the relation of the subject to the great Other[8] but will instead raise the questions of suture and representation.

8. I would like to make a parenthetical remark regarding a certain oscillation in Freudian thought on this subject—which seems to have confused the commentator Strachey in the *Standard Edition* (22:65). The expression "der Träger des Ich-ideals" is translated as the vehicle of the ego ideal, a function of the superego. The term *vehicle* raises some questions. It is in no way necessary to see it as an image of

THE PROBLEM OF SUTURE

Leclaire challenged Miller regarding this inferred suturation. The question remains: Does the suture exist or not? Is not the privilege of not having to suture the indication of the psychoanalyst's position with regard to truth? *How is one to deny that there is a suture when there is concatenation?*

The evidence rests in Freud's much-neglected discussion of the consequences of castration. If castration is possible, if the threat is realized, the subject is deprived of masturbatory pleasure; but castration also implies the much-feared and henceforth irreversible impossibility of union between the castrated subject and the mother. If we consider castration to be the collapse of the entire signifying system because of the rupture of any possibility of concatenation, we may then understand why Freud sees castration as a disaster causing incommensurable damage. In any case the penis plays the role of mediator between cut and suture.

How can suture take place? As we have seen, Miller showed the ascension of the number zero, its transgression of the bar in the form of the one, its disappearance at the moment of passage from n to n′ which is n + 1. But it is not a bad idea to point out that the logic of an "unconscious concept" has requirements inherent in its formation. Let us quote Freud, as Leclaire does: "feces," "child," "penis" thus form a unit, an unconscious concept (*sit venia verbo*)—namely, the concept of a "little thing" which can separate itself from its own body.

We are substituting, then, for binary oppositions (those offered by linguistics, e.g., the phonologic opposition in which relationships are always posited in terms of antagonistic pairs, as well as

---

mechanical support; rather, in this case, we might bring up one of several clues authorizing us to consider a conception of the subject of the unconscious as *Entzweiung* (splitting). The function of the Ideal (*Ideal-funktion*) seems to be crucial here, going far beyond the status of a function; it can best be understood in relation to what Freud aptly terms "the major institutions" (*SE* 14:233), which characterize an instance, in this case the ego—given that which functions within it as a *testing of reality* ("A Metapsychological Supplement to the Theory of Dreams"). This function of the Ideal could be described according to the notion of these "major institutions."

the opposition formulating the basis of all information) *an operational process with three terms (n, +, n') in which each term disappears as soon as it has presented itself.* We end up with a kind of *paradigm* which may lead the way toward what might well be the resectioning (*découpage*) of the signified.

Indeed, linguists run into great difficulties as regards *resectioning of the signified*, whereas the resectioning of the signifier does not seem to give them any problems. Martinet, for example, makes the following remark: "As for the term 'semantics,' if it has acquired the meaning which interests us, it is nonetheless derived from a root which evokes not a psychic reality but rather the signifying process—which implies the combination of the signifier and the signified," "a sememe in any case could not be anything other than a bifaced unity."[9]

Here we run into the following difficulty: any direct reference to the signified would destroy the structuralist enterprise, since its entry via the signifier allows it to make the detour necessary for an indirect—relative and correlative—approach. Moreover, and above all, the mapping out of pertinent traits leaves us perplexed at this juncture.

Thus, it is *the structure of the body* which is lacking here as consistent support. For does not our confidence in the stability of pertinent phonological traits ultimately depend on the functioning of the vocal apparatus? Certainly this apparatus is under the control of the nervous system, which explains linguists' fascination with cybernetics. The psychoanalyst alone listens to meaning, within his own context—that is, while keeping in mind the demands of indirect reference, the analyst considers that resectioning takes place on the level of the signified, and that it is this resectioning itself which implies the resectioning of the signifier which renders the signified intelligible. At this point we are confronted by an ambiguity regarding the linguistic conception of the signifier and its psychoanalytic formulation as Lacan conceives it: are they one and the same?

You have of course recognized in this double-faced unity La-

9. A. Martinet, *La Linguistique synchronique* (Paris: Presses Universitaires de France, 1965), p. 25.

can's theorization of the Moebius strip.[10] But wouldn't it be possible to consider that resectioning of the signified, in this metonymic series of the different partial objects, is represented by the phallus—precisely in that it appears, in the form $(-\Phi)$, through its different partial objects? We already know the diachronic succession of these objects—oral object, anal object, phallic object, and so on: these terms, which merely represent the guide marks distinguishing erotic zones, leave room for more complex forms.

This conception might be a compromise between a strict binary system, which leads us to options bereft of tertiary mediation, and another system in which causality is developed as a network—a reticular system, which does away with all oppositional functioning.

Finally, it seems that *the minimal form of this reticular structure is the triangular structure in which the third element is disappearing.* This, I think, is the operation clarified by Miller's commentary.

This may remind us of the diverse forms of relationships presented by the Oedipus complex, in which an opposition, i.e., sexual difference, insofar as it is sustained by the phallus, is in fact inserted into a triangular system and can only be understood in terms of coupled relationships, in which the phallus constitutes the standard of exchange, the *cause* of exchange.

It is to Saussure's credit that he introduced *value* into the principle of language as system, while sketching in the comparison with political economy at this juncture. But having defined this notion, Saussure did not develop it; he did not ask the question of what constitutes value for the speaking subject. Thus suture takes place here, putting value in relief, at stake (*en cause*), without telling us anything about it.

It is here that we encounter the function of cause developed by Jacques Lacan. If, according to Frege, identity to itself allows *the passage from thing to object,* may we not posit that what we have just shown can function as *the relationship of object to cause?* One may conclude that the object is the signifying relationship linking the two terms, the thing and the cause. In this case, we might be faced

10. This theorization is developed in Lacan's seminar (1965–66).

with one of those examples Freud mentions in the controversial article on the antithetical meanings of primal words (*SE* 11), since we know that thing and cause have a common root, with the object as the path for mediation.

Thus, we shall witness the passage from "the indetermined" to "the state of what is or operates," from "that which is in fact" to "that which is of the order of reason, of the subject or of motive," because of the intermediary of the object in that its definition is "that which presents itself visually or affects the senses."[11]

THE PROBLEM OF REPRESENTATION

It seemed to me that Miller paid only fleeting attention to Frege's many references to representation. However, in the passage quoted above, he did preserve the notion of an *alternating movement of a representation and an exclusion.* The function of assembling, of subsuming, allies itself with the notion of a power which puts things together and which, at the expense of a separation (*coupure*)—operating between the assembling power and the thing presented—*represents. It is separation (coupure) which allows for representation.* But here the number zero appears as an object bereft of representation. It is through the very operation of separation that the subject comes forth, or constitutes itself as subject—at the expense of the *object,* it seems to me. As if one could say: the separation (of the subject) is of no importance since the suture (of the *objet (a)*) remains. *Desire's sacrifice of the object* renders this real, so to speak. The loss of the object is of no importance as long as desire survives and extends it. Or something along the lines of: the object is dead, long live desire (of the Other). Demand becomes that which insures the renewed resurrection of desire in case desire would itself be found missing: demand is formulated via the *objet (a).*

The demand that no cause sustains, a cause whose effect is the hole, by which the remainder is confused with the demand: it is in this manner that the fool (the buffoon) Polonius sees the fool (the

---

11. The terms between quotation marks are those used by Littré under the articles *thing* (*chose*), *cause,* and *object.*

madman) Hamlet, suitor to his daughter and uncertain avenger of the dead Father—who will put another father to death, the father of the object of his desire (Polonius) after a "tragic error."

> . . . that I have found
> the very cause of Hamlet's lunacy. . . .
> I will be brief: Your noble son is mad.
> Mad call I it; for to define true madness,
> What is't but to be nothing else but mad?
>
> [*Hamlet*, II.ii. 48–49, 92–94]

And later:

> That we find out the cause of this effect,
> Or rather say, the cause of this defect,
> For this effect defective comes by cause.
> Thus it remains, and the remainder thus.
> Perpend.
>
> [II.ii. 100–05]

The Relationship of (A) to I(A) and the Problem of Representation and Specularization

Lacan strongly emphasizes the fact that the *objet (a)* cannot be specularized: the mirror image he resorts to is neither the image of the object nor that of representation. The mirror image, says Lacan in his seminar on *Identification* (1962), is *another object which is not the same.* It is caught within the framework of a relationship in which the narcissistic dialectic, limited by the phallus operating in the form of lack, is at stake.

However, we have just seen the un-figurable or image-less object represented by the number zero.

What does Freud make of this? If we consider the problem only along the lines of narcissistic dialectic, it seems to me we short-circuit the problem of representation, which leads back to *the object of drive.* Freud designates this object as eminently *substitutable and interchangeable,* which might compensate for the impossibility of escaping from internal stimuli, or what I would call an intermediate procedure between restricted exchange and generalized exchange.

An object of drive must participate in this exchange as the exchanged term; thus, not just any object is appropriate for substitution.

Two problems present themselves at this point. The first is that of the *distinction between the representative of drive and the affect;* the second is that of the *differential distribution of the mode of representation.*

THE PROBLEM OF THE DISTINCTION BETWEEN THE REPRESENTATIVE OF DRIVE AND THE AFFECT

We know that, in Freud's work, the distinction between the representative and the affect is tentative. Often, the drive is confused with the representative and vice versa.* However, in his last

---

Editors' note: Of the two instinctual drive representations, we are accustomed to thinking that it is affect that is confounded with drive (Rapaport, 1960, p. 881) or with the quantity of psychic energy. In the early phase of psychoanalysis the two were not yet differentiated. (Freud [SE 3:60] wrote, "In mental functions something is to be distinguished—a quota of affect or sum of excitation—which possesses all the characteristics of a quantity.") However, here and throughout this article Green uses psychic representative (*Représentant* in French, *Repräsentant* or *Repräsentanz* in German) to refer exclusively to representation in the sense of idea (*Vorstellung*). For the psychic representative in this sense to be confused with drive ("instinct" in Strachey's translation) hinges either on Freud's (SE 14:177) statement that "an instinct can never become an object of consciousness—only the idea (*Vorstellung*) that represents the instinct can," *or* on the ambiguity noted by Strachey (SE 14:111–12) as to whether the instinct is itself "the psychical representative of organic forces" or whether, as in other passages, "we seem to find [Freud] drawing a very sharp distinction between the instinct and its psychical representative."

But if we have in mind what Freud (SE 14:121) called the *"biological* point of view," the two passages cited by Strachey are not contradictory. Both Rapaport (1957, pp. 270–71; 1959, p. 350) and Loewald (1980, pp. 117–19, 126, 129, 132, 135, 208, 326) have stressed that instinct itself is "the psychical representative of the stimuli originating from within the organism and reaching the mind, as a measure of the demand made upon the mind for work" (SE 14:121). Thus "instinct understood as a psychical representative," as Loewald (p. 117) wrote, "is not a stimulus impinging on the psychic apparatus" (as it was "from the angle of *physiology"* [SE 14:118]) "but is a force within or of the psychic apparatus," which then achieves representation as idea of affect. Instincts *represent* organismic stimuli; they are not these stimuli themselves. Ideation and affect *represent* instincts, and neither of the former should be confused with the latter. See H. Loewald, *Papers on Psychoanalysis* (New Haven: Yale University Press, 1980); D. Rapaport,

writings, Freud progressively establishes and emphasizes a distinction (and this is what I propose to take into consideration) in which *the affect takes on the status of signifier*. The proof of this, since 1923, lies in the progressively specific usage of the *Verleugnung*, translated as disavowal (*SE* 19:143); the most precise formulation of this concept is to be found in the article on fetishism (1927) so frequently referred to by Lacan, the article on the splitting of the Ego (1940), and finally, the eighth chapter of *An Outline of Psycho-Analysis* (1940). Freud then develops the hypothesis that perception falls within the jurisdiction of *Verleugnung*, whereas affect falls within that of Verdrängung (*SE* 21:153).

The possibility in the alternating acceptance-refusal of a global operation or of a partial operation concerning one of the terms (perception and affect) is the condition of the differentiated suture of certain conflictual organizations.

Here, starting from this distinction, Freud envisions the *splitting of the ego*: the *Entzweiung* that Lacan valorizes. However, if Freud creates a term equivalent to repression—disavowal, which has the same semantic value—we must probably conclude that if a signifier alone can meet this fate, the affect enters into the same category.[12]

I even think that the definition of the signifier could profitably be completed in light of what precedes: the signifier would then be *that which, at the risk of its own disappearance, must, in order to subsist, enter into a system of transformations in which it represents a*

Seminars on Elementary Metapsychology, ed. S. C. Miller et al., mimeographed (Stockbridge, Mass.: Austen Riggs Center, 1957, 1959); D. Rapaport, "On the Psychoanalytic Theory of Motivation," in *The Collected Papers of David Rapaport*, ed. M. Gill (New York: Basic Books, 1967).

12. I would like to observe that I have given attention to this point earlier in my critique of Laplanche and Leclaire's presentation at the Bonneral Symposium on the Unconscious in 1960. The paper was published in *Les Temps Modernes* 195 (1962), and was discussed by me in the same issue, pp. 365–79. Both paper and discussion were included in the proceedings of the symposium (6th Bonneral Symposium): *L'Inconscient* (Paris: 1966). Representation and affect are two different types of signifiers. Affect has a major aspect as a discharge process, whereas representation is a production entering into a combinatory system of transformation.

subject for another signifier falling within the jurisdiction of the bar of repression or of disavowal, which thus forces it into a fall from its status of being—in its relationship to truth—and it is via this fall that it gains access to the rank of signifier at its resurrection.

It would be of interest to emphasize the correlation of these two modes of signification, each one encompassing the two mechanisms. In the affect one sees only discharge, although it is—and Freud says so, regarding anxiety—a signal (signifier, for us); in the representative, one sees only the signifier, although it is (in Freudian theory) the engendering of a certain mode of production, therefore of discharge (engendered by the very impossibility of discharge).

In *The Ego and the Id,* Freud returns to the question raised with such difficulty in his article on the Unconscious, of the difference between representative and affect. *The specificity of affect is that it cannot enter into combination.* It is repressed, but its specificity as signifier is such that it can be expressed directly—that is, without passing through the connecting links of the preconscious.

In his seminar on anxiety, Lacan elucidated and demonstrated *that which* triggers anxiety, the way in which the id operates when there is anxiety. But I wonder if he fully realized *what anxiety is,* in terms of its theoretical status. I think it would be interesting to consider affect as an original semantic form compared with the representatives, which act as primary semantides;[13] affect would assume a secondary position which would permit it to acquire the status of secondary semantide, of a nature different from that of the representative and doubling the *Entzweiung* by virtue of this difference. We would then have a reduplication of the nonidentity (to itself), given the disparity of the two levels of the signifier.

Contrary to popular opinion, it is very curious to note that *Freud interprets language as that which transforms thought processes into perception,* and not, as one might suppose, that which dissociates itself from the realm of perception and which would belong to the order of thought. Affect presents us with the effect of the erasure of the perceived trace restored in the form of a discharge.

13. These terms are taken from the vocabulary of molecular biology.

What of the representative? Some considerations regarding terminology may be useful at this point. The long-term discussion of whether to call the "Vorstellung repräsentanz" the representative representer, the representative of the idea, or the placeholder (lieutenant) of representation is not without significance. The ideational representative enters into combination, that much we know. And the ambiguity begins here. The representative does not enter into combination as a homogeneous unity identical to itself. Freud's farsightedness in his field consisted in making from the outset the exclusive distinction, present in memories, between perception and memory. Let us remember the role he attributes to reminiscence insofar as it would be what one might call remembrance in the place of the Other, which keeps the presence of its trace, yet risks losing its quality of remembrance if it should happen to be experienced in reality.

THE PROBLEM OF DIFFERENTIAL DISTRIBUTION
OF THE MODE OF REPRESENTATION

Another type of differentiation interests us here, that between word-presentations and thing-presentations—a distinction which is not fortuitous. Since this differentiation is well known, I refer to it only in order to posit the following: *if there is a theory of the signifier in Freud, it inevitably includes the perceived.* This is apparent in the organization of discourse. Its renewed testimony can be found in the text of our analytic sessions—in the analysand's narrative, the secondary elaboration of the dream, the current or resuscitated fantasy, and the image. The question is to determine whether all that really belongs in the category of the perceived.

This representative of representation shows that one cannot reduce its status to that of perception. Once again, we must note that we are dealing not with presentation but with *re*presentation. *The perceived represents only the point of fascination,* the centering effort of specularization, as Lacan would say. That which allows for the function as zero is of the subjective order, whereas that which ascends to take the place of the 1 is the *objet (a)*, provided that we consider it in this differential distribution—in which nonidentity to itself is demonstrated by this disparity.

The economic point of view is illustrated here not only by being put into play as regards the quantitative evaluation of processes, but also by being identified in this differential distribution. *It is the barrage effect weighing on discourse which necessitates not only combination but also changes of register, material, and modes of representation of the signifier.* These mutations aim at accentuating nonidentity to itself not only in the resurgence of the signifier but in its metonymic metamorphoses as well. Metaphor infiltrates even into metonymic continuity.

Freud's opposition of two systems is of consequence: *the identity of perception* operates in one system, *the identity of thought* in the other. Both are pertinent to our concepts insofar as they are related to truth. But the point of confusion and fascination comes from the consideration that perception can offer itself as a field of identity, while identity operates within it according to a register which is not that of the perceived.

This identity is that which abolishes difference as sustained by lack and which is able to materialize in the perceived, similar to the way in which the identity of thought in the order of thought can only operate after the loss of the object.

It seems to me that Lacan's severe criticism of work being done on negative hallucination was not entirely justified. At the most, one can lament the imprecision of reference points in these works. If negative hallucination is this ascension of the zero considered as not originating in representation, then the negative hallucination would fit in the category of the *representative of representation (ideational representative).* Its value is to give support to the notion of aphanisis, which, as we know, played such an important role for Lacan in the footsteps of Jones.

We must also remember the alternative structure Lacan pointed out in Jones's work on feminine sexuality, which probably has wider implications: *either the object or the desire.* The latter would thus provide the model of a subjective structure, in that it implies the mourning of the object and the coming forth of a negativized subject thus rendered capable of desiring. We should perhaps remind ourselves here that the first mode of representation of the subject, the first i(a), is precisely the product of a representation homologous to negative hallucination: the negative hand of the artist appearing in the contour of the painting which delimits its form. We then see how fantasy positions itself, since the function Lacan assigns to it is *to render pleasure capable of desire.* Here, then, appears a form of emergence of a subject who would escape the destruction of the signifying power in aphanisis, since negative hallucination can be produced but as *specularized lack.* Negative hallucination seems to me to be the inaugural link to Freud's conception of narcissistic identification as relating to mourning of the primordial object. It is *the meeting point of separation and suture.*

It becomes clear that this is the same process which grounds desire in desire of the Other, since mourning places itself as intermediary in the relationship of subject to Other and in the relationship of subject to object.

If the (*a*) comes into play among all these forms (one could say it plays with the fascination of the perceived as it passes through these registers) that is because it is—not as perceived, but as *passage of the subject*—the circuit of discourse. In *Othello,* it is the handkerchief which can appear as (*a*). In fact, and here we are witnesses to the effort of fascination of the perceived, it is not so much the handkerchief which is important as its circuit from the sorceress who gave it to Othello's mother (or to his father; both versions are in *Othello*) to its final destination on the bed of Bianca the whore, ultimately revealing to Othello his desire: "My mother is a whore." This must be demonstrated with the help of knowledge, for Othello, like all those who are jealous, seeks confession more than truth.

Is it not thus that we should understand his soliloquy, when he enters the bridal chamber where, in order to make of his wedding night a night of mourning, he will kill Desdemona?

> It is the cause, it is the cause, my soul—
> Let me not name it to you, you chaste stars!—
> It is the cause.

$$[\bar{V}.2.1-3]$$

The function of the cause here ordains the unquestionable perception of his mother's handkerchief in the whore's hands.

In *The Outline of Psycho-Analysis,* Freud stresses the idea that we live in the hope that, as our instruments of perceiving reality become refined, we will ultimately be able to attain certainty regarding the world of the senses. In fact, he accentuates yet again the affirmation that *reality is unknowable* and that we can only allow ourselves the *deduction* of the true, beginning with the connections and interdependencies existing between the various orders of the perceived. This evidently affirms, if such affirmation is necessary, the preeminence of the symbolic.

But Freud's originality was to introduce at the level of the perceived an order, an organization, which shows the way out of the dilemma of appearance and reality, and to substitute for it that of the ideal (*Idealfunktion*) and truth—this pair which functions in the order of the perceived as well as in the order of thought. Repeated confusion of the symbol and the symbolic ought to arouse our attention and prevent us from taking the one for the other.

What then becomes of the *objet (a)*? It exists as a structure of transformation in which the object of desire moves toward a new mutation and in which *it is desire which becomes object.* Through what operation is the intersection of these enumerated forms through the non-identity to self accomplished? I think these forms can be understood according to the two major axes of synchrony and diachrony if we take Freud's theorization as our reference.

1. *In the synchronic axis,* we have a series formed by thoughts, to the extent that these thoughts are unconscious (and here we must distinguish between word-[re]*presentations* and thing-presentations), *affects* (as secondary signifiers), and two other categories which, it seems to me, should enter into consideration given that we observe them only within the analytical situation: I am thinking about *states of the body proper*—depersonalization or hypochondria, and the like, and about all the manifestations related to what the English authors call parapraxias expressing the register of the act (acting in and not acting out).

2. But we can locate still another series *on the diachronic axis,* which is the axis of the succession of oral, anal, phallic objects, and so on. I wonder if it is profitable to include, as Lacan does, the

scopic object and the auditory object in this series or if they do not, rather, participate in this *register of transmission* between synchrony and diachrony that may be located in discourse in the diverse forms of the dream and its secondary elaboration, of fantasy, memory, reminiscence—in short, all the pathways causing synchrony and diachrony to function. The creation of the *objet (a)*, in which desire becomes object and accounts for subjective positions, operates on the basis of this appropriation. I think this non-identity to itself figured by the blank space is linked to the process of erasing the track (*trace*). This is what forces this system into transformation.

Identity and Non-identity to Self: The Death Drive

The signifier reveals the subject but only by erasing its traces, says Lacan. It is here, I think, that the divorce from all non-psychoanalytic structuralist thought is situated: *in the opposition between visible and invisible, in the opposition between perception and knowledge, the order of truth is at stake for us, but only insofar as this truth always confronts the problem of the erasure of traces.*

Freud says in *Moses and Monotheism* (1938): "In its implications the distortion of a text resembles a murder: the difficulty is not in perpetrating the deed, but in getting rid of its traces" (*SE* 23:43). However, it is in this process that, starting with these traces, makes it possible to go back to their cause, that we find the very process of paternity. In *Moses and Monotheism,* repeating a remark made at the time of the Rat Man article, Freud recalls that maternity is revealed by the senses while paternity is a conjecture based on deductions and hypotheses. The fact of giving priority to the cogitative processes over sensory perception "was heavy with consequences for humanity."

If Freud established a very close tie between the phallus and castration, between sexual curiosity and procreation, it seems strange to me that he never explicitly related the role of the phallus in procreation, its role in the child's desire to have a child, and its role in sexual curiosity.

That which functions on the subject's level as cause (in the search for truth as the question of origins, the relationship to the progenitor) functions as Law on the socioanthropological level. *Here also combination enters into action only under duress of the rule.*

To the prohibition of incest, the interdiction seen and known by everyone which eliminates mother and sisters from the choices in order to indicate other objects in their place, is added the funerary ritual which establishes the presence of the absent one, the dead Father. This is a double process of separation and suture. Among the living, separation from the mother and suture by her substitutes; among the dead, suture of the disappearance of the father by the ritual or totem consecrated to him, separation from him effected by the inaccessible beyond where he is henceforth located.

We have here a striking example of *the separation between Lévi-Strauss and Freud,* illustrated by an unexpected encounter.

Regarding the mask,[14] Lévi-Strauss insists on its simultaneously negative (involving dissimulation) and positive (involving access to another world) function. But for him it seems to be a question of homology, of a correspondence such that in this bifaced reality nothing whatsoever is lost on the way. One might ask, *What is it that necessitates dissimulation,* what forces this structure into a double operation?

Lévi-Strauss talks about a Kwakiutl Indian mask (*Hamshamtsès*) made of several attached panels which make it possible to unveil, to "unmask," the human face of a god hidden beneath the exterior form of a crow. I am willing to accept his conclusion that "one masks not in order to evoke but, finally, in order to unveil"; however, the unfolded mask shows the human face in what could be interpreted as the back of the crow's throat. It would not be stretching the facts to say that the figure presented here reveals the four quarters of the back (two upper quarters and two lower quarters) to be the four members of a character whose torso is represented by the god's face. The analogy between this representation and the one described by Freud in an extremely short text, "A Mythological Parallel to a Visual Obsession," is striking.

14. "Entretiens avec Jean Pouillon," *L'Oeil,* no. 62 (February 1960).

Freud describes an obsessive representation which comes to haunt the patient by way of the name *Vaterarsch,* imagined as a character consisting of a torso and its lower parts, its four members, lacking genitals and head, and with a face drawn on its belly.[15] Freud concluded by positing a connection between the *Vaterarsch,* the arse of the Father, and the patriarch, given that the subject, like all obsessives, displayed filial veneration toward the author of his days.

It seems to me that what is lacking in Lévi-Strauss's work is this sacrifice of the head and genitals represented in the Kwakiutl mask, which exceeds the relation of showing or hiding, but which reveals *the relation of the unveiled to the effaced, to that which has been barred, to lack.* The cause of desire is here.

Freud points out metonymy in the representation of the body substituted for the lack of one of its parts, the genitals. The value of all this is to open our eyes to Freud's interest, at the end of his life, in Moses—not only as a Jew, but also because monotheism appears to be closely tied to the forbidding of idolatry and the complete erasure of any sign of God's presence other than in the form of the Names of the father (Yahweh, Elohim, Adonaï). Here again we notice the redoubling of non-identity to itself.

The work of the death drive, always silent, is localizable in this reduction (in every dimension of the word) which attempts to always reach the point of absence wherein the subject links its dependence to the Other, by identifying itself with its own erasure. The mutation of the signifier, its epiphany underlying its polymorphous and distributed forms, indicates the leap it intends to oppose—as in a dream—to this annulment, and its effort to immortalize itself, profoundly travestied and modified, as witness.

Must we see here, yet again, a marked characteristic of Judaism in its silence regarding the afterlife? The two facts may be connected. But in order to understand the logic of the erasure of the trace, perhaps we ought to give our attention to other temporal-

---

15. This suggests the heads with legs and the Gothic *grylle* figures which G. Lascault pointed out to me. (Cf. J. Baltrusaitis, *Le Moyen-Age fantastique,* ch. 1.)

spatial categories than those with which we are familiar. Perhaps we ought to see here the structures of time and space that the pre-Socratics alone revealed to us, directly or via the analyses of Vernant and Beaufret, each in a very different fashion; but in both, surprisingly, we find indications that the analytic cure provides us with the privileged access to this time and this space, these places and this memory in the Greek sense of the word.

The (a) is revealed in the structures of the nosography to be an episemantic organization and in the modes of the analysand's discourse, which is semantophoric. Here analysts have a passage through a narrow doorway. The approach of structural psychoanalytic technique seems to me necessarily based on the differentiation of representatives and affect and on the differential distribution of representatives.

When reading works on psychoanalytic technique, one is struck by the *total lack of material regarding all that concerns the modes of the analysand's discourse*. However, we do know all the considerable difficulties of cures which do not follow Freud's established model of free association. What is lacking most often is this differential distribution of modes of representation which bears witness to the non-identity to itself of the signifier—the necessary condition for analysis. (I am mentioning this point only as a potential field of research, since I am unable to pursue it further here.)

The essential difficulty in psychoanalytic investigation has to do with its being an *enforced discourse:* it implies on the part of the analysand not only communication, but saying everything. This discourse is a stream of words—*verba volant*—that, unlike the linguist or ethnologist, the analyst cannot shut up in a box. The analyst runs after the analysand's words. Although the death drive infiltrates the analysand's words, in the silence toward which it is always pushing him, the analyst has to deal with living words: living because of their refusal to be reduced to silence, living because of their rebellion against any embalming in which the text is conditioned to lend itself at last to all treatments to which the men of knowledge would submit it.

We will know exactly what (a) is when we will have covered the field of subjective positions. We will then have a vision corresponding to that of the philosopher reflecting on history and culture by means of the modes of discovery of the movement of ideas, of art, of the science of his time—but as a polymorphous, heterogeneous milieu in which diverse forms of alienation are displayed. But let us not delude ourselves. The psychoanalyst, here, is not disposed to abandon his priority to just anyone in the testing of these facts. At the risk of being called imperialist, he will always come to attention before Freud's affirmation that religions represent humanity's obsessional systems, just as diverse philosophies represent humanity's paranoiac systems. Both are esteemed in that they allow the subject to feel superior, says Freud, for having escaped desire and successfully installed something else in its place. And we would have here, in the order of projections of psychic functioning, the first elements of a mimetic conception or theory of the subject's functioning. Psychoanalysis has not yet exhausted the resources of mimesis.

It is insufficient to attribute a function of demystification allowing the conservation of a purged, purified *cogito* to psychoanalysis. It is in fact because Freud starts with dross, detritus, *faux pas,* that he discovers the structure of the subject as relation to truth. This truth is perhaps farther from the image of Prometheus banished for having stolen the fire than from that of Philoctetes abandoned by his kin on a deserted island because of his stinking wound.

REFERENCES

Freud, S. *Standard Edition of the Complete Psychological Works* [*SE*]. London: Hogarth, 1953–74.
"The Neuro-Psychoses of Defence" (1894), vol. 3.
"The Antithetical Meaning of Primal Words" (1910), vol. 11.
"Instincts and their Vicissitudes" (1915), vol. 14.
"The Unconscious" (1915), vol. 14.
"A Metapsychological Supplement to the Theory of Dreams" (1917), vol. 14.
"A Mythological Parallel to a Visual Obsession" (1916), vol. 14.
The Ego and the Id (1923), vol. 19.

"The Infantile Genital Organization" (1923), vol. 19.

"Fetishism" (1927), vol. 21.

New Introductory Lectures on Psycho-Analysis (1933), vol. 22.

Moses and Monotheism (1939), vol. 23.

An Outline of Psycho-Analysis (1940), vol. 23.

"Splitting of the Ego in the Process of Defence" (1940), vol. 23.

Lacan, J. *Écrits: A Selection.* Translated by A. Sheridan. New York: Norton, 1977.

Muller, J., and Richardson, W. *Toward Reading Lacan: Pages for a Workbook,* ch. 6, "On a Quotation Preliminary to Any Possible Treatment of Psychosis," *Psychoanalysis and Contemporary Thought* 2 (1979); 377–435.

Wilden, A. *The Language of the Self.* Baltimore: Johns Hopkins University Press, 1968.

9

From Freud's "Other Scene" to Lacan's "Other"

Antoine Vergote

Lacan's teaching begins with a vigorous "return to Freud." He takes a position at the center of Freudian theory: deciphering the unconscious and defining its status. In opposition to a retrospective Freudianism that presents a diagram of acquired knowledge, he retraces the path of Freud's discovery, not to immobilize it in a literal recapitulation, but rather to keep it alive by bringing a thoroughly cultivated sensibility and an ongoing analytic experience into contact with it. Lacan especially believes that Freud was not in a position to articulate his science of the unconscious because he did not have the linguistics of Saussure and Jakobson at his disposal (*E.*, 799/298).[1] Paradoxically, his return to Freud leads Lacan to make the decisive declaration: "The unconscious is not Freud's; it is Lacan's."[2] As usual, an ambiguous formulation! Does the Lacanian unconscious offer a more rigorous articulation of the Freudian unconscious? Does Lacan better express what Freud meant to say? Or does his concept of the unconscious profoundly transform Freud's doctrine?

Lacan's free pursuit of Freud, at the margin of his thought—hence, in certain respects in opposition to it—is not a question of

Translated by Thomas Acklin and Beryl Schlossman.
1. The letter *E* in parenthetical citations stands for Lacan's *Écrits*. The first page numbers refer to the publication in French, and the number following the slash (/) is the page of the reference in translation. If only one reference is given, it is the French one, meaning that the cited text is not yet published in English.
2. *Ornicar*, January 1977.

analytic orthodoxy but of truth regarding the matter he intends to consider: the unconscious. So my contribution will not be an inventory of Lacan's ideas but a confrontation of his concepts with those of Freud, and within this intermediary space, the conceptual object or focal point will be the unconscious.

Lacan intends to refute any confining interpretation; he nonetheless encourages a retracing of his itinerary: "I always shine beacons so that one can follow the line of my discourse."[3] In fact, throughout his diffracted recapitulations, pedagogical precautions, glimmers or discoveries, or poetic incantations, Lacan always insists on the same conception of the unconscious. Certainly Lacan's thought is an inquiry in progress. But throughout his continual attempts, one essential idea has imposed its presence to such an extent that Lacan puts even the "antecedents" of his theory into the "future anterior": "They will have anticipated our insertion of the unconscious into language" (*E.*, 71). The early Lacan anticipates the later, and the later Lacan is not unknown to the earlier. Just as the witticisms of which he is so fond produce sparks in one's mind rather than being produced by it, so he is possessed by an idea rather than possessing it.

I will therefore dispense with reviewing the mutations of his thought in order to proceed directly to his concept of the unconscious. Whether he presents it in its clinical nakedness or clothed in mythological robes, philosophical livery, or theological chasubles, it is fundamentally the same concept. From his initial return to Freud to his extraordinary declaration "Lacan invented the unconscious," there is a movement which, far from disavowing itself, confirms itself and returns to itself. In Lacan's famous formulation "The unconscious is structured like a language," the words "structured" and "language," more than the "like," gain greater and greater ascendancy over Lacan's thought, whereas Freud, supposing that this formulation is applicable to his thought, tirelessly stresses the disjunction that the "like" opens up.

3. *Scilicet*, 2/3, 1970 (Paris: Seuil), p. 13.

Unconscious Signifiers

The thesis that the unconscious is structured like a language includes two interdependent principles. First, it affirms that the contents of the unconscious consist in elements of language. Lacan regularly designates them with the linguistic term "signifiers." Second, according to this thesis, because of their linguistic nature the contents of the unconscious are organized and transformed according to the laws of language—those described by rhetoric; according to Lacan, these laws are classified in terms of the two axes analyzed by Jakobson, the metaphoric and metonymic axes. The nature of the unconscious, composed of elements of language and structured according to its specific laws, founds Lacan's theory of lack and of desire, which radicalizes what Freud put forward as the search for the satisfaction of wishes. But Freud's wish fulfillment is the law that dominates the primary processes, and the primary processes are those functions which are not governed by the laws of language.

For Lacan, then, the unconscious is composed of elements of language that he assimilates as the signifiers of linguistics (*E.*, 799–801/298–99). Given this conceptualization of the unconscious, his theory presents a double difficulty requiring reflection. It undoubtedly refocuses psychoanalysis on an object that is essential for Freud—that is, the specifically psychic content of the unconscious; nonetheless, for Freud language belongs to the preconscious and to the conscious, a psychic system separated from the unconscious by the bar of repression. On the other hand, Lacan transforms the linguistic concept he adopts, not only to adapt it to the psychoanalytic domain but also to correct a crucial point of linguistic theory. And since these transformations and displacements of the concepts of psychoanalysis and linguistics are not stated in systematic expositions, it is often quite difficult to disentangle objective references from the revisions which set the quoted theory adrift; citations affected by a coefficient which distances them from references deliberately turned into instruments of a new thought.

Freud speaks of "unconscious thoughts." For Lacan the unconscious speaks: "It [the id] speaks." Both formulations show what takes place in analysis: the particular situation of analysis lets the unconscious open up and allows the subject to give a living voice to unconscious representations. In order for this to happen, the unconscious must be *psychic* in the full sense of the word: that which can manifest itself in speech. Lacan's great contribution is that he renewed psychoanalysis by insisting that the unconscious belongs to the domain of language. Upon first estimation, this foundation of Lacan's is actually specifically Freudian. Freud compares the interpretation of dreams to the translation from one language into another, to the solution of a rebus, to the decoding of hieroglyphics. The "dream-thoughts" do indeed consist in a text. And, just as in conscious language, words recovered in more or less ideographic figurations can fill the function of a "determinative" (*GW* 2–3:326/*SE* 4:321).[4] To recount a dream, to track down the narrative through the associations which its elements evoke, to interpret it through successive readings of its polysemic elements, is to give utterance to the unconscious. Does that mean that it speaks? For Freud it only thinks; more precisely, it dreams because it does not know how to speak.

Actually, for Freud it almost speaks. It is insofar as the dream-thoughts are reworked and travestied that they can come forth on the dream-stage. In the dream-formation, Freud identified four moments which allow these thoughts to express themselves in disguise: condensation, displacement, considerations of representability, and secondary revision (*GW* 2–3:511/*SE* 5:507). Only the last of these is "a psychical function which is indistinguishable from our waking thoughts" (*SE* 5:489). In secondary revision— that is, through the labor of the laws of language—dream-thoughts take on an intelligible appearance, but for Freud, "this meaning is the farthest away from the true signification of the dream." Is this not to say that to the extent that it speaks, it is in order to disguise the true unconscious thoughts? Freud nevertheless affirms that unconscious thoughts produce a text that, to a certain extent, can be decoded. He concludes chapter 6 of his

4. *GW* refers to Freud's *Gesammelte Werke; SE* refers to the *Standard Edition.*

Interpretation of Dreams with this decisive affirmation: "Two separate functions may be distinguished in mental activity during the construction of a dream: the production of the dream-thoughts, and their transformation into the content of the dream" (*GW* 2–3:510/*SE* 5:506).

To translate a text, to resolve a rebus, to decode hieroglyphics: Lacan takes these expressions to the letter. Freud's thought lends itself to this, for, at least in his *Interpretation of Dreams,* he compares dream-thoughts to a text which the dream-work deforms, at the same time attributing to that work the apparent readability of a dream. This antinomy can be explained by the novelty of his discovery. In order to affirm the fully psychic status of the unconscious, Freud paradoxically insists upon its relationship to the conscious. He maintains that the unconscious is so entirely "thought" that he will wonder at several junctures what else is needed for thought to become conscious.

Apparently, Lacan's thesis is clear and simple: a text is made of signifiers. This expression has worked like magic on its hearers and it circulates like a password. In its application to the unconscious, however, this concept strangely complicates things. The inflection it gives to Freud's thought is accompanied by a displacement of the meaning which that term has for Saussure, from whom Lacan takes it. According to Saussure's conception, the signifier, originally the acoustic image, is indissolubly linked to the signified (concept, idea). Their relation constitutes the sign, the basic unity of language, consequently defined as a system of signs. From all evidence, the linguistic concept of sign cannot be simply applied either to the dream or to the symptom, since the relation of significance between unconscious thoughts, on the one hand, and on the other hand, the manifested symptom, the dream images, or the dream words which express those thoughts is then broken. Dream images are not signs in the linguistic sense, since their apparent meaning does not correspond to their real meaning.

This is why Freud speaks of two texts. If one wishes to assimilate unconscious thoughts to the kind of language which the translation or the resolution of a rebus reestablishes, it is then necessary to add that this language clings to the signifiers that mask it. Freud calls "signs" the manifest content of the dream. From the point of view of linguistics, this usage is accurate, for it is the manifest dream that contains a residue of true language, utilized by the dream-work to give it an intelligible façade. However, the meaning Freud attributes to the term "sign" is more general: it is the perceptum which manifests something else that is its truth. Consequently, he no longer uses the term to designate the original "text." He does not use the latter expression at all. He never identifies unconscious thoughts with an ensemble of words. The expression "translation" is only a comparison that is used to emphasize the idea of interpretation. Likewise, in his theoretical texts, Freud employs the term "inscriptions" in order to stress that remembrances fixed in the memory are of the order of unconscious thoughts.

If we take the Freudian comparison of translation in its literal sense, we would have to say, in linguistic terms, that we are dealing with two levels of signs composed of signifiers and signifieds. But that would imply denial of the difference between conscious and unconscious. In adapting linguistic terminology in reference to the disguising of dreams, one could say that the manifest signs of the dream are the signifiers and the dream-thoughts are the signified, since the interpretation, according to Freud, reveals precisely the signification of the manifest dream. If, on the contrary, the accent is placed on the dream-thoughts insofar as they are inscriptions in the psyche, then *they* must be called "signifiers." Lacan has taken this option. It carries him far or far afield, in his psychoanalytic theory as in his linguistics.

The signification of the dream being identified with signifiers, signs are now called effects of meaning. "Effect" renders explicit the action of the dream-thoughts on the dream signs and expresses the cleavage of the link signifier-signified, which constitutes the sign in the sense of Saussurean linguistics. Lacan marks these two characteristics by the manner in which he transforms the representation of the linguistic sign. What he calls his "algorithm," $\frac{\text{Signifier}}{\text{signified}}$, replaces Saussure's figure $\uparrow \frac{\text{signified}}{\text{signifier}} \downarrow$. The double bar (single in some texts) designates the cut between unconscious and conscious. The inversion which places the signifier over the signified indicates that the meaning produced by the unconscious signifier conceals more than reveals that signifier.

By inverting the presentation of the linguistic sign, Lacan wants to come to terms with a major difficulty of linguistics as well. Although he has some reservations, Saussure tends to accord a relative autonomy to the signified and to conceive of the signifier as its material support: "A series of sounds belongs to a language only when it functions as support of an idea; taken in itself it is but the material for a physiological study" (1964, p. 144). The revolutionary thesis of linguistics consists nevertheless in the affirmation that the idea does not subsist by itself. Independent of signifiers, thought would only be an amorphous mass. Thought can only become signification through the articulation produced by the signifying system. Concepts, lexical or grammatical categories, are accordingly only differential and are thus not determined by their content (1964, p. 162).

The classical example of the names of colors makes this easily understood: the ideas of colors only acquire their relative identity because the signifiers articulate the color spectrum in découpages where each color is conceived in terms of its difference from the others. If this is so, Lacan is right to invert Saussure's representation and to designate the articulating power of the signifier by placing the signifier on top of the signified. The signifier produces the signified by its precipitation in the amorphous flux of representations.

Lacan further accentuates the autonomy of the signifier by writing it with a capital letter. He does not stop there, for he thinks that the topical cleavage of every psyche into conscious and unconscious affects all language. Thus, linguistics imposes its concepts on the interpretation of the unconscious and, inversely, the thesis of the topical structure of the psyche determines Lacan's linguistic theory. The interpretation of psychoanalysis by linguistics and, conjointly, of linguistics by psychoanalysis results in Lacan's cellular formula: $\frac{S}{s}$. The mark between signifier and signified, which in the formula of Saussure underlines the unity of the signifying relation, becomes "a barrier resisting signification" (E., 497/149). Thus, the unconscious signifier substituted for the unconscious thought empties itself of meaning, since it only has effects of meaning insofar as significance crosses over the barrier.

How can we conceive of a language in which the basic unit, the foundation of linguistics as a science of language, has been destroyed? Since our concern is not specifically linguistic, we will not engage in this discussion. Our sole concern here is to see if Lacan's conceptualization gives an account of the analytic experience and if it can guide it. The idea of an unconscious signifier which would produce an effect of meaning in existence or in a dream seems to be a useful formulation, with the condition that one takes it as an approximative and descriptive language. Then the formulation only posits figures in the unconscious, more or less of the nature of language, that anticipate a meaning to come through associations. Similarly, the words pronounced during an analytic session can be called signifiers for, by the mark inscribed in the unconscious, they are linked together with various chains of unconscious representations and are found to be overdetermined by them in their significations. In analysis, the "signifiers" of language are thus interpreted in the sense of "words," as Lacan let slip from his pen: "A word is not a sign but a knot of significations" (E., 166). It is a question of letting concatenations be produced in which the "signifiers" (words) are unconsciously caught up and which they bring with them when the subject in analysis submits to the fundamental rule of free association. Surely it is never that simple, for such a conception of the cure ignores resistances, a concept which is practically absent from Lacanian theory.

Let us recapitulate. In order to clarify the ambiguities of Saussure, Lacan accentuates the articulating function of the signifier in language and, as a consequence, he inverts the formula of the sign. Interpreting unconscious thoughts as elements of language which do not, however, reveal their meaning, he does not call them signs but rather signifiers separated from meaning by a double bar. Because of the universal topical structure of the psyche, he imposes his "algorithm" $\frac{S}{s}$ as the elementary cell of all language. Whatever the problems that this conception entails for linguistics, Lacan's formulation has the happy result of restoring one of its theoretical and technical elements to psychoanalysis. This formulation revalorizes and justifies free association since it founds it, first, on the power of unconscious representations to anticipate and articulate meaning, and second, on the nature of pronounced words, which in effect are knots of signification. These two founding principles can be expressed in the following ambiguous formulation: signifiers produce effects of meaning.

However, it will be necessary to ask to what extent the Lacanian conceptualization can still sustain Freud's enterprise—that is, the recovery, through the interpretation and the labor of unraveling the dream-work or the symptom-formation, of the unconscious thoughts which are their significations.

The Rhetoric of the Unconscious

The generalized linguistic formula $\frac{S}{s}$ entails the extension of rhetoric to all language and, conjointly, to all unconscious processes. All language becomes what rhetoric calls a figure. All transformations of unconscious representations, at the moment they emerge into consciousness, the body, or behavior, become metaphors. Consequent to the logic of his linguistic formulation of the unconscious, Lacan intends to offer a general theory of significance to linguistics and a strictly linguistic interpretation of unconscious processes to psychoanalysis.

Taking up Jakobson's famous distinction between the two axes of language, paradigmatic and syntagmatic (1971, p. 16), Lacan distinguishes in "discourse"—most of the time identified with language—between metaphor on the one hand, or "word for word," and metonymy on the other hand, the connection by contiguity of signifier to signifier, or "word to word" (E., 506/156). The classic example of catachresis, thirty sails for thirty boats, illustrates metonymy for him; this example, he says, is actually the elision of a signifier, that of the boat. This elision marks "the lack-of-being in the object relation" (E., 515/164). In other words, the hole in language which would like to cover up the being of the

object. No concatenation of signifiers ever really grasps ex-
haustively the being of the object. Thus, all discourse is metonymic. It refers us from signifier to signifier, in an endless path in
which the reference to the object is abolished. The real is thus
"the impossible."

Putting aside the rapid liquidation of the problem of reference,
a problem essential to the philosophy of language, let us examine
the logic of Lacan's thought. Once he has established the unconscious as an ensemble of signifiers and introduced the topograph-
ical cleavage in all language, he must cut off referential relation,
since the unconscious signifier is in fact cut off from its relation
with the real. Consequently, there is no longer any difference
between language (*langue*) and "discourse," spoken language
which bears upon the real to which it refers. It is often objected
that Lacan has introduced concepts in his theory of language
which usually serve to describe the particularities of spoken language. This objection fails to take into account that the logic of his
theory leads him to suppress the distinction between language
and discourse. Moreover, his conception of the subject is connected with this intentional confusion between the characteristics
of discourse and those of language, between the concepts of linguistics and those of rhetoric. Actually, the subject of discourse is
fundamentally the subject of "modern game theory" (*E.*, 860).
The subject is but the locus of the combinative production of
autonomized signifiers. The clinician might even wonder if this is
not the nonsubject of schizophrenia, the one who is the stake of
the word but who is no longer playing the game of language.

The universally metonymic structure of language-discourse,
by undoing the structure of reference to the object, by condemn-
ing the real to be the impossible, is that which makes manifest the
"maintenance of the bar—which, in the original algorithm,
marked the irreducibility in which in the relations between signifier and signified, the resistance of signification is constituted"
(*E.*, 515/164). Lacan's critique of an analysis moving to reestablish
an "object relation," or repair the relation to the real, is autho-
rized by this metonymic conception of discourse.

Via the metaphor, unconscious signifiers can cross over the bar for a while. In opposition to metonymy, which signifies the maintenance of the cut between conscious and unconscious, metaphor as the substitution of one word for another explains the effect of meaning that the unconscious signifier produces. For Lacan, the overdetermination characterizing the dream representation and the neurotic symptom represents the structure of metaphor. As always, he at the same time universalizes "the metaphorical structure" in order that it characterize all production of signification. If all conscious life conceals an unconscious and if the unconscious is made of signifiers, all significance is metaphoric, since every signifier of conscious discourse is a substitute for an unconscious signifier. Once again, the argument is circular. Psychoanalysis provides the model for the theory of metaphor and the linguistic analysis of metaphor grounds the analytic interpretation. There is evidently no reply to such an argument if it effectively accounts for the phenomena in question.

Lacan rightly adopts the contemporary conception in which metaphor, far from being a stylistic embellishment, is a production of new meaning. Even if, in opposition to Lacan, one judges the perception of resemblance to be a constitutive element of metaphorization, it cannot be reduced to a simple comparison; the term *comparison* is inadequate, since no preliminary term contains the signification that metaphor produces. By then identifying all significance with metaphorization, Lacan intends to resolve in one fell swoop the linguistic problem of the proper meaning of words. His answer is simple and peremptory: there is no proper meaning, since all significance is the effect of the substitution of one signifier for another. This idea of a generalized metaphorization is further supported by the notion of the overdetermination of words by their contextual connotations: "There is in effect no signifying chain that does not have, as if attached to the punctuation of each of its units, a whole articulation of relevant contexts suspended 'vertically,' as it were, from that point" (*E.*, 503/154).

Beyond the problematic nature of this conception of metaphor, the important thing here is to find out what becomes of analytic interpretation in Lacan's theory. Is there anything left to interpret if everything has the structure of metaphor, the symptom (*E.*, 528/175) and the dream (*E.*, 515/164) as well as poetry and ultimately any signifying speech whatsoever? Yet this is indeed what Lacan proposes and is what is justified by his definition of metaphor: "The implantation in a signifying chain of an other signifier, by which that which it supplants . . . falls into the ranks of the signified, and as latent signifier perpetuates there the interval in which another signifying chain can be grafted" (*E.*, 708). Certainly the effect of signification, in poetry as in the symptoms, manifests "a crossing of the bar" (*E.*, 515/164), and in both cases there is a latent signifier upon which another signifying chain can be grafted. Yet one does not interpret a symptom in the same way as a poem! As "signifier," the symptom supplants a latent signifier without its falling into the ranks of the signified, at least as long as it is not elucidated. In the poetic metaphor, on the contrary, the substituted "signifier" is actively signified by the metaphoric signifier. The immediate readableness of a metaphor is precisely the outcome of the production of meaning. The symptom, on the contrary, requires interpretation because the sense it produces on the surface is in fact a non-sense of which the hidden sense must be recovered.

At first sight, Lacan confuses the symptom and the interpretation indicating of what "repressed signified" (*E.*, 280/69) it is the signifier. To dream of a wolf, to be seized with panic before a man whom one unconsciously takes to be a wolf, is not *to say*, "The man is a wolf." In a nightmare, the wolf who furiously pounces on the dreamer is but a wolf. At the moment when associations reveal the figures he represents, he can become a metaphor in a sentence which explains the identity of those for whom the wolf of the dream has been substituted. One could say that the dream sometimes employs previously used metaphors, but it de-metaphorizes them, and makes a designative sign out of an action. In metaphor, the metaphorizing term always functions like a predicate (even if it does so implicitly), with the exception of precisely those reused metaphors, which are then no more than vain stylistic ornamentation, as in, "The king of beasts is asleep." These remarks clearly suppose that a distinction is maintained between language and discourse, and that discourse is understood to be the spoken statement (*énoncé*) in which the metaphorical term is associated with a designative sign in the position of subject.

Lacan wants to subvert this common conception because it contradicts the thesis of the universal bar, which, according to him, cleaves conscious from unconscious signifiers and makes all conscious meaning the effect of an unconscious signifier.

Following Freud, Lacan wants to show that every symptom is symbolic. One goes beneath its manifest surface to allow its latent signification to be produced. Freud sometimes arrives at the interpretation of a symptom by clinging to the literality of the word that designates it. This is essentially the case with hysterical symptoms, in which the suffering body symbolizes an unconscious representation through a somatic conversion. Many obsessional symptoms do not have this symbolic structure. But can it truly be said that the symbolic symptom is a metaphor? In addition to the preceding observations, I must still point out that quite often the word that supports "body language" acts as what Freud calls a "verbal bridge." The polysemic quality of the word permits one meaning to be substituted for another and allows for the anchorhold in the body of meaning which is precisely not that of the repressed representation.

Yet the identification between symptom and metaphor is not innocent. It leads to the neglect of the work of interpretation, precisely because of the emphasis it places on the crossing over the bar, whereas Freud insists on the concealment and distortion of the unconscious representation for which the symptom is substituted, although the symptom allows this unconscious representation to appear indirectly at the surface. If the idea of the symptom-metaphor is really taken seriously, one can let the analysand go on "discoursing," convinced that the unconscious signifier will continue to cross over the bar. Freud was already disturbed by the obstinate silence of certain analysts. What is then to be thought of the silence of those who believe even more firmly that "it speaks"?

This confidence that "it speaks" challenges certain Freudian texts on wit (*Witz*) upon which Lacan comments with particular fervor precisely because the unconscious effect manifests itself in the lucky finds of the joke (*Witz*). "There we are," Lacan writes, on "the frontiers at which slips of the tongue and witticisms, in their collusion, mesh together" (*E.*, 801/299). He sees there the evidence that in "the intra-said of a between-two-subjects . . . the transparency of the classical subject is divided and moves toward the effects of 'fading' that specify the Freudian subject which is hidden by an ever purer signifier" (*E.*, 800/299). Are we really dealing with the same unconscious in the witticism and in the slip of the tongue? Freud sometimes seems to mix them together. Yet he never would say of the slip of the tongue, "Anyone who has allowed the truth to slip out in an unguarded moment is in fact glad to be free of pretense" (*GW* 6:116/*SE* 8:106). On the contrary! The slip of the tongue is a symptom, whereas the witticism is related to metaphor. Moreover, most of the time the slip of the tongue calls for a work of interpretation, for it is "the pure signifier" making its irruption in discourse, as an erratic element that must be replaced in the repressed signifying chain. The witticism, on the other hand, refuses interpretation since, just like metaphor, it is sustained only by the interaction maintained between two signifying chains. What is unconscious in the witticism is furthermore not a repressed representation but at most a repressed intention. Analytic practice which confuses the two would speak a word from time to time in order to light, by a quasi-metaphorical play on "signifiers," the spark of a witticism.

Psychic Time

Lacan's considerations on psychic time are singularly illuminating as regards his concept of the unconscious. They concern two phenomena which he links closely together: the effect of meaning of the traumatic event and the organization of the libido.

Freud never elaborated a comprehensive theory of the evolution of the personality, for he was too aware that different factors control several lines of evolution: successive yet not exclusive investments of particular erogenous zones, types of object relation, the effect of repression in the passage from one stage to another, the occurrence of a traumatic event, and so forth. Under the influence of genetic psychology, and even more of the ego psychology according to which the ego takes form progressively as an independent variable, many analysts have tried to establish a genetic history of the libido, punctuated by successive stages. A teleology would thus dominate its development, which would normally evolve from partial drives in relation to a partial object toward integrated drives in relation to the genital object. In a biologizing language that identifies drives with instincts, this genesis is even conceived as an instinctual maturation sustained by a biological scheme.

In returning to Freud and in purifying him of every trace of biologizing thought, Lacan affirms that the "instinctual stages" are organizations of subjectivity "grounded in intersubjectivity" (*E.*, 262/52–53). In other words, they are purely historical. This is fundamentally because, as a being of speech, man pledges his body "in the position of a signifier" (*E.*, 803/301). Refusing the "abject" biologism that has been attributed to Freud, Lacan even interprets the death drive, introduced by Freud in 1920, as "that margin beyond life that language gives to the human being by virtue of the fact that it speaks" (*E.*, 803/301).

The "supposedly organic stages" are thus "particular events of a subject's history" (*E.*, 260/51), comparable to events which stand out as landmarks in the history of a nation. At the moment they take place, they already take on a certain meaning and are already censored in certain respects. Subsequent events can reanimate their meaning, otherwise they erase themselves; their inscription remains alive all the while in the impenetrable archives of the unconscious. When the antecedent event is reproduced after the fact in the external or internal forum by events which recall it, it undergoes a new historicization. Thus the events mesh with one another and are continually transformed through their exchange of meaning. This history is not centered. Time is discontinuous and reversible, for a signifying summary of its moments depends on the meaning that has the upper hand due to the effect of the actual event. No law or paradigm governs the overall course of either a collective or an individual history. All events, including the stages, are accordingly overdetermined in several ways, by their summaries or recapitulations afterward and by the dialectic between the recapitulations and the censorship that expunges or distorts the chapters of their history.

Since the essential form of discourse is an address to the Other and since what is sought in speech is the response of the Other, every event, insofar as it is a historicization, refers to the discourse of the Other (*E.*, 298–99/85–86). Accordingly, the historicization of stages and events consists in the meaning that they are given in view of the expectations of others and not in the recording of events by an objective eye turned toward the past. "What is realized in my history is not the past definite of what was, since it is no more, or even the present perfect of what has been in what I am, but the future anterior of what I shall have been for what I am in the process of becoming" (*E.*, 300/86). In referring to the discourse of the Other, one places oneself in an anterior moment (the future anterior) in relation to one's own future project, since the Other is always ahead of that future. We can then understand one of Lacan's celebrated formulations: the unconscious is the discourse of the Other. By his speech, which evokes, desires, or prohibits, the Other stamps memories with the seal of pleasure and stamps events forced out of memory with the seal of shame or suffering.

It is incontestable that in elucidating the organization of the libido and the impact of traumatic events as a history instituted by temporalizing and intersubjective speech, Lacan powerfully revived Freud's essential ideas. It can be doubted whether he attributes to organic modifications the importance Freud gives to them and which, for him, partially account for conflicts and repressions. The thesis of the primacy of the signifier in relation to historical inscriptions places the accent upon the soliciting discourse of the Other.

The unconscious is the discourse of the Other. But what is this discourse? The Other is itself found to be under the sovereignty of language. The subject and the Other find themselves, in their discourse, at the interior of a language that is preordained. This means that the synchronic structure of language dominates the

ANTOINE VERGOTE   209

historical time of discourse. The future anterior ultimately refers
to the atemporal synchronicity of language. For it constitutes the
essential structure of language: however "more hidden . . . it is
this structure that takes us to the source" (E., 805/303). In the
syntagmatic dimension, the signifiers are linked in discourse in
such a way that each term anticipates the others and the others
determine the meaning of the preceding ones by their retroactive
effect; this is the historicity established by language. Yet, as we
have seen, meaning is produced by "metaphor," which, by substituting one signifier for another, operates in the synchronic
structure. However, according to Lacan, the real cannot bring
about this substitution. Thus there are always gaps of meaning
which are not filled in. The unconscious as "discourse of the
Other" is then without a doubt essentially composed of the immense clamor of language which the subject anticipates in addressing himself to the Other, but which remains inexorably outside consciousness in the future anterior of language. Here one
of the chief ideas of the "structuralist" current of thought can be
recognized. One could compare the conception I have just presented with the hypothesis of Lévi-Strauss, for whom the myths
and rites of a community are fragments drawn from a stock of
mythemes and rites that no group, nor all groups taken together,
can achieve, but which are available in the structure of the unconscious.[5]

Thus, the individual unconscious is formed within a network of
language, made up of family and cultural myths, of appeals and
responses, of desires and interdictions. That which is repressed is
a moment of history. Yet history is a discourse about an event, a
retroactive discourse overdetermined by various events after the
fact, further overdetermined in its possible significations by its
reference, in the position of the future anterior, to the discourse
of the Other, which is itself overladen with language, "the signifier's treasure" (E., 806/304). Language as the supraindividual
domain of signifiers is the middle party which envelops the in-

5. J. Lacan, Le séminaire, livre XI (Paris: Seuil, 1973), p. 23. See also Lacan, The
Four Fundamental Concepts of Psycho-Analysis, p. 20.

terlocution between two subjects. Thus Lacan's definition: "The unconscious is that part of the concrete discourse, insofar as it is transindividual, that is not at the disposal of the subject in reestablishing the continuity of his conscious discourse" (*E.*, 258/49). Or, again: "Since Freud the unconscious has been a chain of signifiers that somewhere (on another stage, in another scene, he wrote) is repeated, and insists on interfering in the breaks offered it by the effective discourse and the cogitation that it (this discourse) 'informs'" (*E.*, 799/297). For Freud as well, the unconscious is rooted in a collective history. The Oedipus complex and all that is tied up with it, the birth of culture, of morality, and of religion, derive from prehistoric events which *Totem and Taboo* tries to reconstruct. Yet while Freud founds the genesis of mankind on a battle of strength, Lacan supposes that at the outset it was language, law, and symbolic pact, preordained, which made mankind.

The two definitions of the unconscious that I have just cited do not mention repression resulting from a conflict. One could think that Lacan does not linger over what is self-evident. Actually, for Lacan, the unconscious is already present as a cut in conscious discourse, because only a few echoes of discourse or of transindividual human language reverberate in consciousness; furthermore, we will see that this discourse is not the discourse of man nor of historical humanity, inasmuch as it is "the treasury of the signifier." The unconscious is thus composed of all that is lacking in "omnicommunication" of the "omnipresence of human discourse" (*E.*, 265/56). The subject is split from the moment he enters into language, divided between his conscious discourse and the omnidiscourse that envelops and overlays him.

This division is indeed more essential to Lacan than the stories of repression. Caught up in the transindividual chain of signifiers, the subject is at each instant only the incidence upon him of a signifier that refers to another signifier. When he speaks, he *is*, insofar as a signifier makes its irruption in him. Thus, telepathy is nothing but the coincidence in two subjects of the same signifiers that flow in the communicating networks of the unconscious. Thus, we see that the confusion on Lacan's part of slips of the tongue and witticisms is not a failure to recognize the distinction between unconscious and preconscious but the hypothetical affirmation of an unconscious essentially defined by the presence and the effect of chains of autonomous signifiers which appear in bits and pieces in the flickering of consciousness. "The register of the signifier is instituted from the fact that a signifier represents a subject for another signifier. This is the structure of dreams, slips of the tongue, witticisms, of all formations of the unconscious. And it is this which explains the original division of the subject" (*E.*, 840).

An essential part of Freudian psychoanalysis is the work on resistances and the tracking down of repressed mnemonic representations. Psychoanalytic practice that attempts to be consonant with Lacan's theory will not give these the same importance. The secondary repressions upon which Freud's analytic work has its bearing are no more than occasional events in which the primary repression, in Lacan's sense, is tangibly accomplished: the omnipresent failure of recognition (*méconnaissance*) inherent in consciousness itself. As soon as man speaks, he has already lost himself: "Being of non-being, that is how I as subject comes on the scene, conjugated with the double aporia of a true survival (*subsistance*) that is abolished by knowledge of itself, and by a discourse in which it is death that sustains existence" (*E.*, 802/300). A veritable "subsistence," this is the unconscious as chain of signifiers. This unconscious opens for a moment, in the finds of witticisms, in dreams, in symbolic symptoms, even more clearly in deliria. But what man speaks and what he thinks is but "the trace of what must be in order to fall from being" (*E.*, 801/300), a trace that must be such that it knows that its discourse stirs up nonbeing (or nothingness) and that the conscious I is but a semblance of being. "Substance" is the Other, the chain of signifiers.

The Other

What Lacan sees as the effect of meaning of unconscious signifiers can be summarized: conscious discourse and symptoms are the tropes (metaphors and metonymies) of their movement.

His linguistic inversion of the relationship of signifier-signified and his psychoanalytic generalization of metaphor already indicate that his "unconscious" no longer has the same signification as Freud's. To relieve the term of its duplicity, it is necessary to consider the principle upon which Lacan founds his original understanding of the unconscious. I shall willingly call his fundamental principle a metalinguistics in the sense Freud intends in elaborating a metapsychology that should replace metaphysics. The term *metalinguistics* signifies, then, that there is no beyond of language and that the entire metaphysical tradition finds itself demystified by its reduction to language. Second, what I call metalinguistics is substituted for Freud's metapsychology in that Lacan replaces the concept of the economy of instinctual drives with the movement of signifiers. Many inquiries about Lacan and his relationship to Freud remain unresolved because these bases of his thought are left in the shadows. His art of covering over his ideas with subtly diverted citations and commentaries, moreover, spreads confusion. Is this a strategic cleverness or the spontaneous rhetoric of a generalizing metaphorization? Or both? It matters little.

Lacan's thought moves within the great tradition of philosophy and is developed on the horizon of theological culture. But he settles accounts with them by a subversion which retains their "symbolic structure" while reducing their content and intention to a surface mirroring—in a word, to the imaginary.

Analytic experience illustrates, for Lacan, the knowledge of ancient wisdom of religion and philosophy: that man does not possess his own discourse, because this discourse finds itself under the motion of a truth which surpasses it. "It speaks" in man, for even if he has the illusion of leading his own discourse, in fact a truth leads him he knows not where. Metaphysics linked the domain of knowledge to that of truth and thought truth to be superior, insofar as all knowledge participates in it without ever coinciding with it. Furthermore, the rationalism invoking Copernicus deludes itself by positing a center of the cosmos, and that invoking Darwin deludes itself with the belief that men are "the top dogs in creation" (*E.*, 797/295). The ecliptic, judged to be a naive representation, would in fact furnish "a more stimulating model of our relations with the true" (*E.*, 797/295); it would signify the reference to a symbolic system which dominates knowledge and ordains the articulation of time.

Nor does man have his desire at his own disposal. The unconscious wishes that Freud discovers in dreams and in neuroses are but the fragmentary manifestations of a fundamental movement which leads man on without his being able to master it. Lacan gives the name *desire* to this movement, reminiscent of the Platonic Eros and of "natural desire" in Christian metaphysics. Within this tradition, desire constitutes the essential dynamism of the human being; it is called natural insofar as it is anterior to and yet underlying all particular tendencies, precisely because it is rooted in him by his divine origin.

Hegel takes up this tradition and rationalizes it. He offers the philosophical model that is at once homological with and antithetical to the Freudian revolution as Lacan intends to pursue it. On the one hand, Hegel, like Freud, refuses the false evidence of feelings and lived experiences; he defines in them the coordinates at the interior of a logic. On the other hand, his "epistemogenic" logic tends to reabsorb all representation, to elevate it to the level of concept until it reaches the achievement of consciousness in self-consciousness by its conjunction with absolute knowledge, thus suppressing the difference which is primary for metaphysics between knowledge and truth. For Lacan as for Hegel, a secret reason underlies knowledge and desire, but "the dialectic that sustains our experience (as analyst) obliges us to understand the ego from beginning to end in the movement of progressive alienation there where self-consciousness is constituted in the phenomenology of Hegel" (*E.*, 374).

Lacan prefers to return to "the rationalism that organizes theological thought" (*E.*, 873), which teaches us the structure of the relation of the subject to truth as cause. In fact, in the beginning, theology posits "language," or so Lacan subversively interprets the "Logos" at the beginning of the fourth Gospel.[6] Everything—

6. J. Lacan, *Le Séminaire, livre II* (Paris: Seuil, 1975), p. 325n.

the human body, the world, human discourse—is thus the effect of the original letter. As for theology, human life is inscribed in the book of God "in quo totum continetur" (in which all is contained), for Lacan all is contained in the treasury of the signifiers-causes. But these do not refer beyond themselves. "God is unconscious" (xi 58/59; see note 5); this is "the veritable formula of atheism" and of the Lacanian unconscious. To affirm God is to want to close the chain of signifiers upon a center, whereas it only operates by the absence of a center, by its essential lack (*E.*, 819/317). To posit God would moreover be to endow the signifiers with a reference and a meaning, the two coinciding for Lacan, whereas they are only the causes whereby sense is manufactured out of non-sense. Lacan exalts some elements of Saussure's linguistics to the transcendental level. Signs (which have become signifiers, and we have seen why) are purely differential; they form a closed ensemble, and reference does not define their linguistic entity. Their closure does not, however, suppress movement, for there is the essential hole of the lacking signifier, that of the phallus, a lack which inexorably marks discourse and human desire with a lack that Lacan calls symbolic castration.

Thus, one should interpret the formulation "it speaks" to the letter, for the unconscious is man caught by the letter of signifiers without signification, which preexist at the beginning and which come to be localized in him. The philosophical or religious quest for meaning is but the vain wandering of man who does not know of what cause he is the effect. Psychoanalysis is not, like religion, a question of meaning, but of structure (see the letter Lacan published in the Paris newspaper *Le Monde*, 11 January 1980, p. 19). There is no meaning; there is only the causality of the scriptural signifier, to which man is consigned for the wandering of his desire and thought, having for its object only something which is nothing (*E.*, 498/150). Yet the poetry of nothingness is not vain; in collecting seminal letters, in submitting to them rather than directing them, in allowing them to operate their diabolical art, man and woman experience enjoyment. The enjoyment (*jouissance*) of female mystics is paradigmatic. They think they are enjoying God, the substantial Other of religion. Lacan, stripping religious rationality of its imaginary rags, interprets: their enjoyment is that of the Other, the "of" having the sense of subjective genetive, and "Other" the sense of the chain of signifiers.[7] This is why "the essential testimony of the mystics is precisely saying that they are experiencing it (enjoyment), but that they know nothing of it." It (Id)—or the Other—enjoys in them.

The Unconscious: Chain of Signifiers or Unlettered Underworld?

The "it speaks" substitutes the metonymic chain of signifiers for the anonymous, wild energy of the id, which in his second topography Freud borrowed from Groddeck (1923). This substitution is such an important subversion that it authorizes the declaration that "Freud did not invent the unconscious; Lacan did." The "subtle body" (*E.*, 301/87) of language, in effect, expels from the psychoanalytic field the concept of instinctual drives, that hard core of Freudian theory. How then is the dynamic unconscious to be understood as that part of the id that is repressed? What do we make of the Freudian difference between the (pre)conscious, which is the domain of language, and the unconscious, which, lacking language, is not governed by its laws? This question posits the entire problem of a psychoanalytic cure, since for Freud healing takes place in a lifting of repression when words come to repressed representations. And what remains of the Freudian theory which characterizes psychosis as the abolition of thing-presentations such that word-presentations, cut off from the original history of the subject, no longer refer to the real and words are treated as things? Does clinical experience verify the pertinence of Freudian theory or that of Lacan?

For one who reads Lacan's letter to the letter, the ultimate goal of psychoanalysis must be to bring to recognition the nothingness unveiled in the hollow of the letter, and to release from it a poetry of enjoyment (*jouissance*). To heal from meaning is not as such a goal that can be pursued. This goal, more than any other, can be reached gratuitously, or in addition. Here Lacan rejoins the paradoxical path of Buddhism. And as in Buddhism, he intends his

7. J. Lacan, *Le séminaire, livre XX* (Paris: Seuil, 1975), pp. 70–71.

radicalization of antihumanism to conjure up the suicide that tempts those who, alienated by semblances of meaning, obstinately continue their vain quest for them.

Lacan's theoretical apparatus has contributed greatly to restoring to speech its therapeutic force in analysis. The accent placed on the textuality of the unconscious, first of all, heightens attentiveness to the overdetermination of words, to the incorporation of the letter in certain forms of bodily suffering, and to the grammatical structure of drive vicissitudes. If analysts forget that psychoanalysis moves within the field of language precisely because man is a speaking being, they will be tempted to guide themselves "by some supposed 'contact' experienced with the reality of the subject" (*E.*, 252/44). Or else, boasting that they go beyond Freud's technique, still considered to be rather awkward, they center the analysis on the feelings experienced here and now in the analytic relationship, on what is called an "analysis of the transference." Others take the struggle against resistances to be the axis of therapy and make the analysis into a duel. By reminding us that symptoms have the structure of language, Lacan has liberated psychoanalysis from that which falsifies the analytic dialogue: the active intervention of the analyst, the explanation of the neuroses as caused by certain events, the pursuit of objective memories, the effort directed toward an introspective awareness. . . . The refusal of a beyond of language has a positive consequence: it condemns the prejudice that leads to an inquiry into the truth of the circumstantial evidence. What is important is to verbalize the events, to make them "pass into the *verbe,* or, more precisely, into the *epos* by which he brings back into present time the origins of his own person" (*E.*, 255/46–47).

The critiques of psychoanalysis which inaugurate various schools of therapy, such as those of Perls or of Watzlawick, all rest upon failures of recognition that echo those current in the teachings of the analysts themselves. The most common is the identification of the speech of the cure with the theoretical explanation of the symptoms. The cure is then degraded into "a 'causalist' analysis that would aim to transform the subject in his present by learned explanations of his past" (*E.*, 251/42). In promoting the idea of the unconscious "structured like a language," Lacan first of all wished to restore to speech as verbalization all its power of historicizing and structuring remembrance.

This said, too quickly, it remains for us to consider the displacements and inversions to which Lacan has submitted Freudian concepts. Lacan's unconscious is not Freud's, since for Freud the unconscious has the nature of *not* being like language. Indeed, I earlier indicated Freud's ambiguous statements that initially served to support Lacan's theory. But while Freud progressively elaborates his idea of the unconscious precisely in order to conceptualize its differential status, Lacan takes the opposite direction and his discourse on the unconscious wants to come forth like the discourse of the unconscious itself. This progressively greater divergence from Freud cannot be without its effect upon analytic practice. One may even wonder if, at the point where his theory is pushed toward its consequences, we are not witnessing a new occultation of the unconscious. The fascination that Lacan exercises over literary circles ignorant of clinical realities recalls the misunderstanding between Freud and the surrealist poet André Breton. The theory of a universalized rhetoric offers the radically negative mysticism that some literary devotees or those nostalgic for an impossible ecstasy of madness are looking for. Yet how can the work of psychoanalysis be conceived according to such radically transformed theoretical coordinates? The least that must be said is that, in Lacan's discourse, the clinical references have become fewer and fewer, and more and more evasive. That in any case ought to incite us to make a new return to Freud, beyond Lacan, while bringing along with us what we have learned from him. The important thing here is to question the aporia that clinical experience imposes on Freud: the unconscious is a psychic reality precisely insofar as, being liable to resolution through interpretation in speech, it must be akin to language; yet it remains unconscious insofar as it is not structured like a language. Freud's efforts to adjust his concepts to the clinical experience of the unconscious lead him to elaborate a theory of an immense complexity. The summaries offered by manuals or those in opposition to psychoanalysis read like parodies. This reminder of the essential elements will only serve to show what is problematic with Lacan's unconscious.

According to Freud, a *kind of* unconscious functions *like* a language and unconscious contents are *in part* composed of inscriptions in the psyche of marks which are *like* words. This is precisely the unconscious resulting from secondary repression, upon which psychoanalysis can labor, the unconscious which nevertheless does not really have its place in Lacan's theory.

First, the mode in which the unconscious functions presents some similarities with rhetorical processes. These are the "mechanisms" of the unconscious: the displacement of affect, the condensation of representations, the somatic conversion which makes a bodily symptom into a symbol, obsessional isolation. These can respectively be compared to the litotes, to the composition of characters in a novel, to an expressive symbolic act, to analytic fragmentation or eventually to the institution of a symbol. The unconscious visibly borrows its processes from thought regulated by language; but that is in order to escape from thought. Let us consider the first process cited—displacement. Even in the earliest studies, Freud notes the essential difference between the rhetoric of the unconscious and that of the conscious. "The *hysteric,* who weeps at [the representation] *A,* is quite unaware that he is doing so on account of the association A—B [the really sad memory], and B itself plays no [further] part at all in his [conscious] physical life. The symbol has in this case taken the place of the *thing* entirely." Freud opposes "normal" symbolism to hysterical displacement, which produces the unconscious symbol. "The knight who fights for his lady's glove *knows,* in the first place, that the glove owes its importance to the lady; and secondly, he is in no way prevented by his adoration of the glove from thinking of the lady" (*SE* 1:349).[8] Thus a signifying intention animates normal symbolization. The unconscious, however, takes up its structure (*GW* 2–3:346/*SE* 4:340) so as to eliminate the signifying intention. If this intention is constitutive of symbolism, it follows that the unconscious desymbolizes the symbol.

8. This Freudian text has not been included in *GW*.

Consequently, the entire Freudian theory is necessary to interpret it. But in opposition to the symbol, the unconscious "symbol" disappears whenever it is translated into signifying language. The Freudian technique is correlative to the concept of the unconscious as destructuration of language.

Yet this destructuration serves the intention, unconscious to be sure, to cut off the reference to memories that are too painful. The force of instinctual drive runs counter to their investment, without being able to prevent the affective energy from seeking, in spite of everything, an unconsciously expressive outlet in the unconscious symbol. Thus, the functioning of the unconscious as a reversed usage of the structure of language can only be understood by introducing two related concepts: an economic one, psychic energy; and a linguistic one, reference. Yet these are the two concepts Lacan expels from his theory of the unconscious and of language. Thus, his theory does not seem to account for metaphor, the normal symbol, or for the unconscious. It is impossible to understand how significance is produced by crossing over "the bar," by what process the repressed defends itself against a translation into language.

Lacan is certainly right to maintain the linguistic nature of certain unconscious contents. After his contribution, it can no longer be possible to assimilate the unconscious to primary needs, to instincts of a biological nature, or to the destructuration of conscious content operated by psychophysiological conditions. Whatever the ambiguity of the term *signifier*, it designates a type of unconscious content. When Freud pursues the lifting of repression at the moment of sudden awareness, it is indeed a matter of mnemonic representations which belonged to previously inaccessible archives. The irruption, in the case of hysterical psychosis (*GW* 1:62, 88–89, 93/*SE* 3:38), reveals a certain unconscious content that normally remains repressed or only comes forth masked in dreams and in neurotic symptoms. One can call "signifiers" the signifying representations that compose this unconscious. Yet I would prefer Saussure's term *sign* specifically because, in these cases, the signified is indissociable from its signifying support. The suspension of reference, which determines the confinement of delirium, allows signs (Lacan's "signifiers") to turn like luminous rings. This unconscious is structured like a language, yet it does not function like a language in the act of "discourse." But in the repressed unconscious, it is the functioning of the unconscious which utilizes the proceedings of language borrowed from rhetoric.

Thus, the unconscious is never simply structured like a language. Freud's entire theoretical effort aims to conceive simultaneously of the similarity and the dissimilarity between the unconscious content and functioning on the one hand, and language on the other. This is why some of his texts contradict each other. His metaphors of translation or of the rebus point out the similarity. His more theoretical texts insist on the cleavage. For Freud, language defines the structure of the preconscious in opposition to the unconscious. The latter is said to be deprived of all that characterizes language: time, causal links, the intention to communicate. . . .

This tension in conceptualization is not simply the result of a theoretical difficulty. It corresponds to a layering in the unconscious as well. Certain contents, nearer to the preconscious, are more structured by the laws of language. Other, more archaic ones are less organized by language. They are, I believe, those Freud calls "thing-presentations" in opposition to "word-presentations" (*GW* 10:294–303/*SE* 14:196–204). Thing-presentations are not the same as representations of things. In the latter expression, the "of" has the meaning of the objective "of," referring to the things which are represented, whereas by thing-presentations Freud suggests the form of presentations, as in his expression *Sachbezetzungen der Objekte,* thing-presentation of objects. These are presentations that, unlike words, are not referential signs. These presentations thus have the nature of a thing. They are the first investments of objects, as the expression indicates: thing-presentations of objects. These presentations are the condition necessary for language to function as language, which no longer operates in psychosis because of the abolition of thing-presentations, the supports of object investment. Thus, for Freud, it is the language of the psychotic that would be composed of pure signifiers, slipping without anchorage because they lack reference to objects. Interpreted to the letter, Lacan identifies the unconscious with psychotic language, which, according to Freud, lacks precisely the unconscious support necessary for it to function as language.

Lacan teaches us to hear in the analytic "discourse" the future anterior as well as the restaging of memory, the reserves of signifying virtualities as well as the displacements which deform. I have read and listened to his discourse in that manner, with a fervor that has not allowed itself to be alienated. It has seemed to me that he is right twice over: in promoting the return to Freud, and in finally declaring that his unconscious is not Freud's.

REFERENCES

Freud, S. *Gesammelte Werke*. London: Imago, 1942.
———. *Standard Edition of the Complete Psychological Works*. London: Hogarth, 1953–74.
    The Interpretation of Dreams (1900–01), vols. 4, 5.
    Jokes and their Relation to the Unconscious (1905), vol. 8.
    Totem and Taboo (1913), vol. 13.
    Beyond the Pleasure Principle (1920), vol. 18.
    The Ego and the Id (1923), vol. 19.
Jakobson, R. "Two Aspects of Language and Two Types of Aphasic Disturbances" (1956). In R. Jakobson and M. Halle, eds., *Fundamentals of Language*, 2nd ed. The Hague: Mouton, 1971.
Lacan, J. *Écrits*. Paris: Seuil, 1966. *Écrits: A Selection*. Translated by A. Sheridan. New York: Norton, 1977.
———. *The Four Fundamental Concepts of Psycho-Analysis*. Translated by A. Sheridan. New York: Norton, 1978.
Saussure, F. de. *Cours de linguistique générale* (1915). Paris: P.U.F., 1964.

Lacan in Use

10

"The Universe Makes an Indifferent Parent": *Bleak House* and the Victorian Family Romance

CHRISTINE VAN BOHEEMEN-SAAF

> Our solitude has the same roots as religious feelings. It is a form of orphanhood, an obscure awareness that we have been torn from the All, and an ardent search: a flight and a return, an effort to reestablish the bonds that unite us with the universe.
> —Octavio Paz, *The Labyrinth of Solitude*

> Our classifications will come to be, as far as they can be so made, genealogies; and will then truly give what may be called the plan of creation. . . .
> Light will be thrown on the origin of man and his history.
> —Charles Darwin, *The Origin of Species*

I

The following reading of *Bleak House* is an attempt to combine a Lacanian approach toward narrative structure with a cultural-historical outlook in the light of Cesare Segre's conclusion in *Structures and Time* that a "definition of narrative models must be arrived at from within a study of cultural modelling systems."[1]

This essay on *Bleak House* is part of a longer discussion on family romance and the novel, *The Plot of the Novel from Fielding to Joyce*.

1. C. Segre, *Structures and Time* (Chicago: University of Chicago Press, 1979), p. 56.

The narrative model informing *Bleak House,* both Esther Summerson's story and the third-person narrative, is a version of the family romance. While the story of the orphan who finds his parents, or a home, is a perennial literary theme, the ways in which this process of discovery or rediscovery are imagined differ from period to period, and may be a symbolic expression of the deepest, often unconscious notions of human identity and destiny. Here my argument will be that the peculiar structural shape of Dickens' family romance may also be detected in a contemporary, nonliterary text, in fact positivist in inspiration, that of Darwin's *Origin of Species,* and can be seen as a reflection of the cultural tensions of the epoch.

As my point of departure I have selected a quotation from Paz's *The Labyrinth of Solitude* which situates "orphanhood"—the inevitable separation from a full presence—as a metaphor for the human condition as experienced in the modern era. At first sight this term may not seem to apply to *Bleak House,* which presents itself as a story about the corruption of Victorian society, especially the law. The plot traces the fates of those who have had the misfortune to deal with the Court of Chancery, and focuses upon the personal history of Esther Summerson, who is ignorant of the identity of her parents. As we shall see below, orphanhood, as loss of parents, loss of origin and identity, not only applies to Esther but also summarizes the thematic and structural concern of *Bleak House.*[2]

2. The aesthetic theory which supports this view, and on which this analysis is based, is related to the work of D. W. Winnicott, Marion Milner, Hanna Segal, and others, who are often grouped as the "object-relations school" of psychoanalysis. For a recent exposition of the contributions of this school to an understanding of the creative process, see A. F. Marotti, "Countertransference, the Communication Process, and the Dimensions of Psychoanalytic Criticism," *Critical Inquiry* 4 (1978): 471–91. Marotti argues that "object-relations psychoanalysis provides psychoanalytic criticism with better models for creativity and aesthetic response than the classic notion of sublimation. Placing the child's relationship to the mother at the center of psychoanalytic theory, it concentrates attention on the self-other transactions of infancy that shape identity, establish modes of relationship with the environment, and lead to the attainment of individual autonomy" (p. 477). However, Hans W. Loewald argues in "The Waning of the Oedipus Complex," in

Let us begin, then, with defining that aspect of the Darwinian solution which is of importance with regard to *Bleak House*. John Dewey once summarized Darwin's achievement in the following way:

> In laying hands upon the sacred ark of Absolute permanency, in treating the forms that had been regarded as types of fixity and perfection as originating and passing away, the *Origin of Species* introduced a mode of thinking that in the end was bound to transform the logic of knowledge, and hence the treatment of morals,politics, and religion.[3]

Darwin's treatise is based on a revisionary strategy which replaces the older, theologic world view of a *Scala Naturae,* founded on the principle of discrete hierarchical levels and a divine creation ex nihilo, with a biologic, evolutionary understanding of reality, based on the notion of genealogy and natural origin. In terms of the current critical fashion of understanding conceptual structures as tropes, one might say that Darwin attempted to substitute a metonymical or syntagmatic world view for a metaphorical or paradigmatic one; however, since I shall relate Darwin's conceptual strategy to a novel embodying abstractions in the situations and roles of everyday life, I prefer (while aware of the crudeness of this schematization, to which I shall return later) provisionally to summarize Darwin's strategy as the dislodgement of God the Father by Mother Nature as the locus of origin.

To the modern reader, even one raised in a fundamentalist environment, it may be difficult to realize the unsettling power of Darwin's suggestions about origin. After all, thinking in biological terms has become a natural habit to us; but much of what we hold as obvious truths—for example, that a human body is made up of cells, that conception entails the penetration of an ovum by

---

Papers in Psychoanalysis (New Haven: Yale University Press, 1980), that the Freudian concept of the Oedipus complex should be seen not as a temporary crisis to be permanently superseded but as a perpetually renewed psychic structure. As so often in the history of psychoanalysis, Freud anticipated his revisionists.

3. J. Dewey, *The Influence of Darwin on Philosophy* (New York: Holt, 1910), pp. 1–2.

a spermatozoon—was still fairly specialized knowledge in our grandparents' generation. Belief in spontaneous generation of some non-human genera was still current, and the baffling phenomenon of biological origin often required the postulation of a transcendental causative agency, a "vis creatix," an "anima" or "entelechy." Our modern understanding of ourselves as sexual beings depends on and testifies to the replacement of a hierarchical world view by an evolutionary, or more precisely, a biological one; and the entrenched nature of our views, which may close our eyes to the pain and profound uncertainty of those who lived through the period of transition, ultimately depends on the explosion of biology as a science during the nineteenth century.[4]

In selecting natural history as the matrix of this conceptual change, however, I do not want to suggest that the shift in understanding was limited to the realm of science. On the contrary, though the general public may not have been aware of all the implications or able to understand the actual processes of scientific investigation, interest in origins and beginnings was in the air. As early as the 1820s a general enthusiasm for natural history and geology arose, kindled by popular lectures, introductory booklets, and so forth. The implications of the geological findings about the age of the earth were widely and eagerly discussed because they conflicted with the biblical account of creation. Even poets concerned themselves with this discussion. Byron, for instance, defends his use of Cuvier's account of the creation in the preface to *Cain* as not contradictory to the Mosaic account. But what captured the popular imagination more than anything else was the discovery of prehistoric monsters. A model of a dinosaur

4. The mid-nineteenth century witnessed the publication of three important theories which led biology to develop fully as a science: (1) Virchow, in *Die Cellularpathologie* (Berlin: 1858), argued that all cells derive from preceding cells; (2) Pasteur disproved the theory of spontaneous generation in bacteria, thus necessitating the conclusion that all organisms come from preceding organisms; (3) Darwin asserted that all species came from earlier species. It was not until 1879, despite the earlier knowledge of the existence of spermatozoa, that Herman Tol, a Swiss physician, actually observed the penetration of an ovum, and invalidated the age-old theory that sperm induced a "spiritual" effluence which effected fertilization.

was reconstructed for the Great Exhibition of 1851, and Dickens' own *Household Words* featured a description of a megalosaurus only a few months before he started working on *Bleak House,* which contains an oddly unexpected reference to that animal in its opening paragraph.[5]

This popular interest in science, this fascination with the primeval, should be regarded as more than a mere desire for novelty or sensation. An element of fearful fascination with the disturbing implications of these findings no doubt played a part in making them so attractive. With the widening realization that man's historical origins are not "divine," and that he is, in this respect, not intrinsically different from the rest of the primate world, the problem of human identity becomes increasingly acute.[6] The best-known contemporary articulation of the deeper feelings of the Victorian public is Tennyson's *In Memoriam,* published the year before *Bleak House* began to appear. I quote the beginning and end of poem LVI, which express the moral threat of the notion of mere biological origin and the poet's agony at having to give up the illusion of superiority to the natural world:

> "So careful of the type?" but no.
>   From scarped cliff and quarried stone
>   She cries, "A thousand types are gone;
> I care for nothing, all shall go."

> "Thou makest thine appeal to me:
>   I bring to life, I bring to death:
>   The spirit does but mean the breath:
> I know no more."

. . . .

5. See S. Shatto, "Byron, Dickens, Tennyson, and the Monstrous Efts," *The Yearbook of English Studies,* ed. G. K. Hunter and C. J. Rawson, no. 6, 1976.

6. I take the difficult term "identity" in its etymological meaning as relating to *idem,* "the same." Finding one's origin, then, is finding out who one is. Cf. the beginning of Martin Heidegger's "The Origin of the Work of Art," in *Poetry, Language, Thought,* trans. A. Hofstadter (New York: Harper & Row, 1971): "Origin here means that from and by which something is as it is. What something is, as it is, we call essence or nature. The origin of something is the source of its nature" (p. 17).

> No more? A monster then, a dream,
>   A discord. Dragons of the prime,
>   That tare each other in their slime,
> Were mellow music match'd with him.
> O life as futile, then, as frail!
>   O for thy voice to soothe and bless!
>   What hope of answer, or redress?
> Behind the veil, behind the veil.

This desperate lamentation about the looming presence of "Nature, red in tooth and claw with ravine" provides an intellectual context to the narrative mood of the opening of *Bleak House*. For all the famous realism of the first paragraphs, which situate the reader in a densely concrete, vividly recognizable London suffering the effects of late autumn weather, the novel's initial descriptive passage is haunted by the same doubts which are expressed in *In Memoriam*. Its unique effect depends on a typical Dickensian strategy: while (re)creating a scene, the narrator presents it in a manner which points up a vital lack of essence, of rigidly circumscribed identity in the object of description.[7] Everything moves, slides, and slithers while staying in its place, not because the narrator would wish us to regard the world under the aspect of process, as modern philosophy might suggest, but because phenomenal reality seems to lack a fixed, definite origin. And without circumscribed origin, there can be no circumscribed identity or shape.

If we look more closely at this description, we see that the shifting and shimmering outline with which Dickens represents London is related to a stylistic peculiarity. The main clauses lack finite verbs, which have been elided. Action is indicated by present participles, and the passage remains in a continuous present. There is an absence of *tense*, suggesting the absence of *time*. In a perpetual present there is no past and future, no beginning or

7. Dorothy Van Ghent discusses the fluidity characteristic of Dickens' descriptions of inanimate objects and the reification of his portrayal of people in "The Dickens World: A View from Todger's," in M. Price, ed., *Dickens: A Collection of Critical Essays* (Englewood Cliffs, N.J.: Prentice Hall, 1967), pp. 26–27.

end, only a perpetual being "in the middest," a sense of uncertainty about what precedes or follows, since the ambivalent present precludes certainty about origin or destiny; and what the narrator primarily seems to want to stress is the absence of a beginning. Thus, when accidentally referring to "daybreak," he hastens to qualify this by adding in parentheses: "if day ever broke" (ch. 1).[8]

It is not surprising to note, therefore, that night and day have become an indistinguishable blur through the supremacy of fog, that the "death of the sun" has effaced the difference between climates and seasons, or that with the collapse of the temporal distinctions, land, sky, and water have turned into an indiscriminate mixture of mud. Placing this opening passage next to its prototype, the story of the creation in Genesis, one is surprised to find that *Bleak House* "creates" its vision of London by the deliberate blurring of precisely those distinctions which in the biblical account had constituted the divine act of original creation—the separation of land and water, darkness and light, and the institution of the heavenly bodies to mark and measure time. While the setting remains London, we seem to have moved to a temporal perspective outside biblical or recorded time, a blend of prehistory and perpetual present which would seem to account for the narrator's disorientation, and the expectation of seeing a megalosaurus on Holborn Hill.[9]

The inability to hear what the narrator calls "the rushing of larger worlds," and to "see them circle around the sun" (ch. 2), is not merely a peculiarity of the beginning of the story. Throughout his account the third-person narrator will betray the deadlock

8. All quotations refer to the Crowell Critical Library Edition, ed. D. DeVries (New York: Thomas Y. Crowell, 1971). This reprint faithfully reproduces the first one-volume edition of September 1853.

9. Most probably it is the notion of mud which suggested the megalosaurus to Dickens. Cf. "Owen's Museum," *All the Year Round*, vol. 8, 27 September 1862, p. 63, which gives the following description of the prehistorical scene: "For the world was not then as lovely as it is now, but huge, and monstrous, and uncouth—a mere seething steaming cauldron of heated mud and turbid water, inhabited by fierce monsters always warring together." It was, of course, still a general Victorian belief that monsters generated spontaneously from mud.

of being bereft of a principle of coherence, a key to make firm sense of things. The world he points out to us is not merely fallen or less perfect than in its pristine state; it has lost its principle of cohesion. In giving up the belief in a metaphysical patriarchal origin, this world has relinquished the cosmographical conception of the Great Chain of Being in which the hierarchical levels were bonded by love. But whereas the informing spirit seems gone, the relics of the older world view, the hierarchical institutions which administer society, live on as fossilized relics of the earlier age. Thus the "raw afternoon is rawest, and the dense fog is densest, and the muddy streets are muddiest, near . . . that leaden-headed old corporation: Temple Bar." While "hard by Temple Bar, in Lincoln's Inn Hall, at the very heart of the fog, sits the Lord High Chancellor in his High Court of Chancery" (ch. 1).

Chancery, then, is the central symbol of the evil aftereffects of this loss of a principle of meaning: instead of justice, this court of law produces endless reams of meaningless writing; rather than providing for the "wards of chancery," the members of this court have made the process of administration self-serving: "groping and floundering" in a moral fog, like the pedestrians of the preceding page they are "mistily engaged in . . . an endless cause, tripping one another up on slippery precedents, groping knee-deep in technicalities, running their goat-hair and horse-hair warded heads against walls of words" (ch. 1). Its most important judge, the Lord High Chancellor, is shown to the reader not as the human representative of the divine prototype whose prestigious power he still shares in the symbolic order, but as the icon of ineffectiveness. Not a "father," not a provider for the orphans of his world, this Lord, lacking the radiance of numinosity, sits at the heart of the moral darkness of the story like the spider in its web, with a "foggy glory round his head," looking into "a lantern that has no light in it" (ch. 1). With a biblical metaphor, chancery symbolizes the death of the "spirit" and the tyranny of the "letter." In this novel crowded with orphans, chancery is emblematic of the absence of God the Father, and cause of the bitterness of Mr. Jarndyce's retort to Skimpole that the "universe makes an indifferent parent" (ch. 6).

The narrator's vision also reflects the nobility as a dead, lifeless institution, crumbling now that its inspiring principle has lost the power to bind. One notes with a sense of irony that the seeds of the impending downfall of the Dedlock family were planted during the reign of King Charles the First when the English Revolution swept aside the notion of the divine right of kings, based, of course, on the sanctity of the hierarchical principle. Though the steps on the ghost walk predicting the event have rung for several centuries, it is during Lord Dedlock's lifetime that the family skeleton, illicit relations with the "other party," brings about the end of the lineage. As Lord Dedlock is the aristocratic counterpart of the Lord High Chancellor, his beliefs and preferences personify the lack of vitality of the social structure. Threatened by the political activity of Mr. Rouncewell, his housekeeper's son, he laments that "the floodgates of society are burst open, and the waters have—a—obliterated the landmarks of the framework of the cohesion by which things are held together" (ch. 40). Here again, the narrator uses the image of flooding water—a traditional symbol of the female, the other, the unconscious—to denote the breakdown of the hierarchical order, an image which will recur just before Esther confronts her dead mother in the wetness of Tom-all-Alone's.

However, what is important here is that Lord Dedlock's fears for the breakdown of the discreteness of the hierarchical levels seem to make him suspect in the eyes of the narrator, who, ambivalently, keeps hammering on the fact that law and aristocracy have degenerated into things of "precedent and usage; oversleeping Rip Van Winkles" (ch. 2), fossils of an earlier world view. It is one of the signs of Miss Flite's madness that she still regards the aristocracy in a mystique of presence—firmly maintaining that it is only the best people who are raised to nobility, whereas the narrator demonstrates over and over again that the relation between essence and appearance, ideal function and social actuality, is lost or lacking. Just as in Dickens' other novels, most notably *Little Dorrit,* in *Bleak House* the social structure is denounced for having made mediation into a self-contained, inescapable way of life. Mr. Jarndyce's perception of this is perhaps the clearest in the novel: "Through years and years, and lives and lives, everything goes on, constantly beginning over and over again, and nothing ever ends. And we can't get out of the suit on any terms, for we are made parties to it, and *must be* parties to it, whether we like it or not" (ch. 8). Without a relation to a fixed origin or end, men are forced to live in a permanent halfway house, or, as Richard Carstone describes his emotional state, "an unfinished house."

This uncertain state entails problems of identity and role. In their inability to bear the provisional quality of their existence, Dickens' characters reach irritably after an illusionary role or strategy to give their lives identity and outline. Some, like Miss Flite, Gridley, and Richard Carstone, believe against reason in a "Last Judgment" which will retrospectively vindicate their sacrifice of human qualities. Mrs. Pardiggle and Mrs. Jellyby are restless in their efforts to enforce or propagate the ministration of Old Law-charity, while neglecting to love their children at home. Harold Skimpole's opportunistic game-playing seems especially telling: unwilling to suffer the disillusionment and diminishment of adulthood, he plays the role of the irresponsible, careless child; the supreme irony is that Skimpole, a parent himself, manipulates the real orphans of his world into providing for him. Another desperately selfish stance is Mr. Chadband's passionate intensity as a preacher. He perverts "truth" into "Terewth," and all moral distinctions are flattened beneath his oppressively vindictive dogmatism. These assertive stances toward life are subterfuges to escape suffering, refusing the knowledge that the better characters in the novel patiently bear, a sense of being left without directive, of being an orphan in a bewilderingly complex world. Though sentimental to modern tastes, it is precisely in his pathos that the figure of little Jo, the orphan, seems to personify the loneliness, the keylessness, and perplexity of most of the inhabitants of *Bleak House*:

> And there he sits, munching and gnawing, and looking up at the great Cross on the summit of St. Paul's Cathedral, glittering above a red and violet tinted cloud of smoke. From the

boy's face one might suppose that sacred emblem to be, in his eyes, the crowning confusion of the great, confused city; so golden, so high up, so far out of his reach. There he sits, the sun going down, the river running fast, the crowd flowing by him in two streams—everything moving on to some purpose and to one end—until he is stirred up, and told to "move on" too. [ch. 19]

Jo's physical and emotional loneliness while looking at the cross, the central symbol of the patriarchal culture which seems to exclude him, stems from lack of education, and marks his separateness from the web of cultural traditions and beliefs which Jacques Lacan has called "the symbolic order." Nevertheless, this inability to interpret the cross, the failure to lend it vital significance, is best read as an ironic displacement of the powerlessness of society at large to find a "key" to unlock a fuller spiritual presence.

Let us explore this idea more fully. French structuralism has enforced awareness of the fact that the tradition of Western culture is founded on a complex of interrelated axiomatic ideas, referred to by Lacan as "phallocentrism," implying that patriarchal power and the prestige of the written word are the operative principles of our social and conceptual structures. In this view, key, cross, gavel, and sword are symbols of the same ordering principle. And what Dickens shows us in *Bleak House* is not just the aftereffect of the "death of God" but the tottering imbalance of this ordering principle, the uncertainty about its continuing effectiveness.[10] Thus when logocentrism (to take a liberty with Lacan's term) threatens to fail, writing eventuates in meaningless documents, or it turns subversive, as in the letters of Lady Dedlock and her illicit lover, which lend a threatening presence to what should have remained hidden or nonexistent, a relationship not sanctioned by logos and law. Similarly, if phallo-

10. The notion of the "death of God," and its importance for nineteenth-century fiction, has been dealt with at length by J. Hillis Miller in *Charles Dickens: The World of His Novels* (Cambridge, Mass.: Harvard University Press, 1958) and in *The Form of Victorian Fiction* (Notre Dame, Ind.: University of Notre Dame Press, 1968). I am indebted to his views.

centrism begins to fail, the traditional relationships within the family break down, especially between parents and children. In addition to Mrs. Jellyby and Harold Skimpole, the patriarchal Mr. Turveydrop, a self-inflated "model of deportment" living parasitically off the labor of his daughter-in-law, is an example. Lady Dedlock, we note with surprise, never rectifies the abandonment of her daughter Esther; whereas little Charley, herself an orphan, must parent and provide for her brother and sister. Relationships between man and wife also become unpredictable: Mrs. Jellyby wields the pen while Mr. Jellyby creeps self-effacingly through the house; Mr. Snagsby lives in terror of his wife, while the Bagnets, a humane couple, play the game of never acknowledging Mrs. Bagnet's superiority to her husband in a pretense of continued conformity, because "discipline must be maintained." Even the most lovable character, Mr. Jarndyce, can no longer assume the power and authority belonging to his place in society. While he emulates divine benevolence, he hides his uncertainty behind the gruffness of a friendly giant. It is only the villain of the story, the lawyer Tulkinghorn, who, as his name suggests (tool-king-horn), does assume full masculine authority.

II

As a novel, *Bleak House* is of course more than a record of the disintegration of our cultural heritage. It would not be a Dickens novel if it failed to offer a solution to the ills and evils it so powerfully evokes; and here we must return to the passage from the conclusion to the *Origin of Species*. Just as Darwin insists that biological research should give up its outdated concern with determining the essential nature of discrete species and study instead the history of their development in order to find "the origin of man" and "the plan of creation," just so Dickens proposes to remedy the evil of a disintegrating hierarchical world view by simultaneously tracing connections on several levels which will ultimately sketch the pattern of a new view of origin.

In the chapter entitled "Tom-all-Alone's" he asks:

What connection can there be, between the place in Lincolnshire, the house in town, the Mercury in powder, and the whereabout of Jo the outlaw with the broom, who had the distant ray of light upon him when he swept the churchyard-step? What connection can there have been between many people in the innumerable histories of this world, who, from opposite sides of great gulfs, have, nevertheless, been very curiously brought together! [ch. 16]

It is in the course of tracing Esther Summerson's illegitimate origin—her "natural genealogy," to use Darwin's phrase—and in neutralizing its unspeakable character that this question is answered.[11] In the process of revealing the secret of Esther's mysterious natural origins, Dickens also sketches the failing links in the crumbling social edifice, however tentatively; he transforms what may initially have seemed a random kaleidoscope of Victorian images into a design, even a meaningful design, because Esther's first-person account will outstay the disturbing vision of the third-person narrator and conclude the story with the assurance of personal happiness, secure identity, pattern, and order, in a pristine little Bleak House.

As narrative, Esther's quest for identity belongs to the genre of romance. Its suggestive power hinges on the diametrical opposition between good and evil, enemy and hero, which is characteristic of the genre.[12] Whereas society at large is associated with "winter, darkness, confusion, sterility, moribund life, and old age"—the romance qualities of the enemy—Esther, and her substitute family at Bleak House, breathe "spring, dawn, order, fertility, vigor and youth."[13] More specifically even, Esther's story may

11. I do not mean to suggest that Dickens' tracing of connections should not also be seen in the light of mid-Victorian literary practice. As Peter K. Garret points out, "the large loose baggy monsters of the 1840's–1870's meant to transcend the limitations of the individual point of view and envision the life of the whole community" ("Double Plots and Dialogical Form in Victorian Fiction," *Nineteenth-Century Fiction* 32, no. 1 [1977]: 1–18).

12. F. Jameson, "Magical Narratives: Romance as Genre," *NLH* 7 (1975): 135–63.

13. See J. I. Fradin, "Will and Society in Bleak House," *PMLA* 81 (1966): 108. The quotes are from N. Frye, *Anatomy of Criticism: Four Essays* [1957] (Princeton, N. J.: Princeton University Press, 1973), pp. 187–88.

be seen as similar to that version of the quest for identity Freud
has given the name "family romance," which revises the actual
circumstances of birth and origin, replacing the unacceptable
real parents with imaginary others of higher social standing.[14]
Though Esther's aristocratic mother *is* her biological mother, and
not the product of a revisionary fantasy, still, Esther's origin is
constructed in the course of the story; and while the reconstruction
is not the revision of the banality of the parents—which, according to psychoanalytic theory, is one of the possible motives for
constructing a family romance—it is the revision of an even more
fundamentally ego-shattering situation, their absence.

When we meet Esther Summerson, she lives in ignorance of the
identity of her parents. An apparent orphan, a "child of the
universe" (ch. 6) as Harold Skimpole euphemistically calls her,
her plight is similar to that of little Jo, even though Esther lives
just within the pale of respectability. In her insecurity about origin, she summarizes the emotional condition of almost all inhabitants of the novel, including the third-person narrator. But as the
plot unravels, Esther is slowly revealed in her true, mysterious
identity: the lonely girl proves to be the daughter of a Captain
Hawdon—alias Nemo—who has died in Krook's house, and Lady
Dedlock, the most beautiful, most fashionable, most repressively
controlled lady in the land. Though on an unconscious level
being the daughter of "Nemo," "nobody," may suggest creation
ex nihilo or grandiose illusions of virgin birth, the name Nemo,
which hides identity rather than revealing it, constitutes their
denial. It is the badge of Esther's illegitimacy. She is born outside
the law, outside the patriarchal order, and as such, her godmother tells her, it would have been better had she not been born
at all. Without a father, she can never be acknowledged by polite
society; she will not inherit a preexisting social identity. Esther's
illegitimate existence is so threatening to the social order that her

---

14. The term occurs first in Otto Rank's *Der Mythus von der Geburt des Helden*,
published in 1909, where Rank incorporated Freud's ideas as part of his own
argument. See S. Freud, "Family Romances" (1909), *Standard Edition of the Complete Psychological Works* (London: Hogarth, 1959), vol. 9.

own mother, even after the existence of her daughter has become known to her, cannot acknowledge her. When she is finally forced to do so, her fall brings with it the towering prestige of the ancient Dedlock lineage.

For this reason this first triangle of the family romance, this first (re)construction of an identity which proves more subversively threatening than its absence, is slowly overlaid and encompassed by a new revisionary triangle, the final one, consisting of Esther, her husband Alan Woodcourt, and the fatherly Mr. Jarndyce, who made it all possible. Esther's story, then, is a double family romance: the narrative practices secondary revision upon its own original (re)construction of origin.

In order to unravel the secret necessity of this curious strategy, we must return to the situation of the first triangle. Freud argues that when the child is old enough to know the sexual facts of life, his family romance will show evidence of the truth that *pater semper incertus est* whereas the mother is *certissima*. The namelessness of Esther's father and the dangerous presence of her mother would seem to conform to this pattern. Moreover, Freud points out, the romance takes on an erotic orientation, motivated by curiosity about the sexual activities of the mother, often projected as illicit. Had we been engaged in an analysis of *Bleak House* as the reflection of Charles Dickens' personal story, our conclusions would have been predictable.[15] However, Dickens' narrative strategy is his answer to a problem which transcends the discretely individual; the absence of the father, the unbridled sexuality of the mother, reflect the threat of the new ideas about the origin of man and the creation of the earth, of a suddenly powerful and prolific Mother Nature, dethroning the ancient figure of God the Father. In the light of Jacques Lacan's reinterpretation of Freud, hinging on the operative dualism of the "Name-of-the-Father" (as the principle of symbolic order) and the opposing "Other" (as territoriality, irrationality, materiality, and the moth-

15. On Dickens' oedipal problems and their reflection in his work, see L. J. Dessner, "Great Expectations: 'the ghost of a man's own father,'" *PMLA* 91 (1976): 436–49.

er), a widely cultural *and* psychoanalytic interpretation of *Bleak House* as family romance would seem to be possible. In other words, if the narrative progresses as a secondary revision of Esther's identity, this is because her illegitimacy stands for the uneasy suggestion of a purely biological, nonphallic, nontranscendental notion of human origin. And this notion must, finally, be repressed from the consciousness of this Victorian novel.

Though the author cannot and will not discuss the symbolic implications of Lady Dedlock's motherhood, its unconscious presence provides the impetus for this long and revisionary narrative. As we shall see below, it is Esther's "quest" for her mother, and the necessity to come to terms with her own female sexual nature, which necessitates the many twists and turns of this fiction. This is seen most easily when we compare the two triangles of Esther's family romance again. The difference in the second is the absence of the mother, and Esther's newly acquired status of married woman—even mother. Would it not have been easier, then, from the point of view of an author constructing his plot, to have let Lady Dedlock die before the story began? This would have obviated the necessity of removing her from the scene in order to suggest a happy ending with greater force. But in that case, what would have been lacking from the novel is its wide social panorama. Indeed, it is Lady Dedlock's sin and its contagious aftereffects, connecting Chesney Wold, Tom-all-Alone's, chancery, and Bleak House, which together produce the panorama of Victorian society for which we especially value the novel. Therefore, the problem of female generativity, though not alluded to in the text, is its central inarticulated nexus and motivating impulse, forcing it through endless visions and revisions to "answer" its underlying question.

Since the overwhelming question remains implicit in the structure of the narrative and is never articulated openly, the importance of Lady Dedlock's sexuality for Esther's accession to her own motherhood is far from self-evident and forces us to scrutinize Dickens' revisionary family romance with an eye to its structural and symbolic ambiguities. It is at the moments of puzzling ambiguity, when the unconscious irradiates the text with its peculiar numinous aura, that the public and the personal, the familiar and the subversive, have been welded together by the poetic imagination. In a text dealing with identity and origin, what better starting point can we select than the ambivalence of its portrayal of Esther's "self"?

Like many other fictions, *Bleak House* represents a character's quest for selfhood in the image of the search for a permanent house or home.[16] In this, just as in her orphanhood, Esther is representative of what moves and motivates the other inhabitants of *Bleak House*, who live in a "Ruined House" (one of the projected titles for the novel), an "unfinished house," or at best, in the disenchantment of a "Bleak" house. Through the analogy of sympathetic magic, Esther's search, leading her from the foster homes of her earlier days to the boarding school of the Miss Donnys, and on to the quasi-permanence of her stay at Bleak House, is redemptive of all the others.

The crucial point, however, is that though at first greatly honored and tempted by Mr. Jarndyce's offer to become the mistress of Bleak House, Esther cannot and must not accept his benevolence. She must move on to her own detached home. It is only after she has been described as happily at ease amidst husband and children, living in a small-scale model of Mr. Jarndyce's Bleak House, that the novel finds its end. It is Esther's assumption of the detached house, then, rather than her renewed beauty or the discovery of her parents, which marks the fulfillment of her quest. Yet the little house is not so detached after all; there is a curious ambivalence in its symbolic connotation which condenses two different—in fact, opposed—aspects of Esther's hard-won identity. Most obviously, as a place separate from the corruption of society, and separate from the fatherly Jarndyce, it would seem to indicate Esther's social, moral, and emotional autonomy. On the other hand, in its odd metaphorical relation to Mr. Jarndyce's house, of which it is the exact replica, down to the most insignifi-

16. Gaston Bachelard states that with "the house image we are in possession of a veritable principle of psychological integration. . . . [It] would seem to have become the topography of our intimate being" (*The Poetics of Space,* trans. M. Jolas [Boston: Beacon Press, 1969], p. xxxii).

cant detail, almost as if houses spawned little ones, Esther's final house would seem to mark her as reproductive, generative, sexual. The little house is also the nest, and we see Esther referring proudly to her own two little girls.[17]

Looking back over Esther's development as a character, one notices that the ambivalence of the final symbol of selfhood has been present in Dickens' portrayal of her all along, and reflects an underlying ambivalence in the novel's notion of human identity. From Esther's earliest moments of conscious reflection, her awareness is structured by the tension between her true but unmentionable natural identity and the necessity to ensure a place and role in the patriarchal social system to which she is an outsider. As she gathers from her godmother's unrelenting insistence that she had better not have been born at all, the anniversary of her birth is a day of evil and sinful disgrace to those sharing the secret surrounding her birth. Esther's manner of coping with the social and emotional isolation of her position is to deny that deepest, most natural part of herself, which in her childish understanding merely seems to keep the "wound" of the day of her birth open. This "natural" self, on which her own generativity and full womanhood depend, she projects upon her doll, the only one to whom she opens her heart. But this child had better never been born at all: departing for school, Esther buries her doll in the garden. Simultaneously, she sets out to win social approval with the vow "to repair the fault I had been born with (of which I confessedly felt guilty and yet innocent) . . . and [to] strive as I grew up to be industrious, contented and kind-hearted, and to do some good to some one, and win some love to myself if I could" (ch. 3). From the very beginning, then, Esther's "self" is split into

17. In *Dickens on the Romantic Side of Familiar Things: Bleak House and the Novel Tradition* (New York: Columbia University Press, 1977), while discussing the notions of "the Uncanny" ("das Unheimliche"), Robert Newsom refers to Freud's view that the home is, ultimately, the mother's womb (p. 61). Although his book is also a study of the "romantic side of familiar things" in Dickens' novel, Newsom does not view them under the aspect of the family romance. He sees "familiar" and "romantic" as opposites, and accounts for the novel's texture in terms of their tension.

two halves, one "buried" and unmentionable, one obsessively concerned with conformity to patriarchal views of feminine identity. We might say that Esther's struggle for selfhood takes place at two levels simultaneously, one questing for an identification with the (m)other in order to achieve sexual identity, the other for substitute fatherhood and a place in society.[18]

Initially, the attempts to earn a place in society and the protection of a father figure occupy the foreground of the narrative. At the Miss Donnys', and then at Bleak House, Esther persistently attempts to blot out the shame of her birth by trying to become an "original" herself. As everyone agrees, she is a model of deportment—a "pattern young lady," as detective Bucket praises her—obsessively creating order out of disorder and stalling the disintegration of society at large (domestically reflected in the state of Mrs. Jellyby's closets) by her unrelenting diligence and the protection of her household keys, which she jingles to the refrain of "Esther, duty, my dear." Indeed, Esther's attempt to lock out the

---

18. The critical view of Esther as a flawed character has lately superseded the earlier indictment of her character as insignificant, hypocritical, or falsely sweet. Alex Zwerdling argues in "Esther Summerson Rehabilitated," *PMLA* 88 (1973): 429–39, that "Dickens' interest in Esther is fundamentally clinical: to observe and describe a certain kind of psychic debility. The psychological subject matter of Dickens' later novels demanded a new narrative technique, in which the character could present himself directly. . . . Esther Summerson is Dickens' most ambitious attempt to allow a character who does not fully understand herself to tell her own story" (p. 432). Though I do not disagree with Zwerdling, I am not here concerned with psychological realism. I focus instead on Esther as a function in a narrative strategy, an "actant" in a story, to use Greimas' term. From this analytical point of view the dualism of Esther's character is related to Taylor Stoehr's findings in *Dickens: The Dreamer's Stance* (Ithaca: Cornell University Press, 1965), which point to the many instances of doubling in this novel. Apart from the two voices and their contrary visions of the world, doubling has led to the creation of many pairs of characters which are "projections onto separate characters of the conflicting impulses of the dreamer. Through them Dickens conveys the ambivalence and complexity of his dream meaning without expressly stating it" (p. 167). Stoehr sees the function of the double plot as keeping social and sexual problems from intermingling. My interpretation differs in that I try to show that on a deeper level, they are concerned with the same ontological problems of identity, but that only the private confrontation leads to the suggestion of resolution.

"original sin" leads her farther and farther away from selfhood to the perfection of an imaginary, obsessive role, and to speaking to herself in the third person; when her substitute father and guardian finally offers to marry her, it momentarily seems as if Esther will become, like her biblical namesake, "a queen" of starry purity.[19]

For all Esther's exertions to earn an unfallen status, at moments of emotional crisis the repressed image of the doll revives in her memory, bringing with it softer sensations. When the young lawyer Guppy proposes marriage in the chapter entitled "Signs and Tokens," her own refusal leaves her perturbed: "I surprised myself by beginning to laugh about it, and then surprised myself still more by beginning to cry about it. . . . I was in a flutter for a little while; and felt as if an old chord had been more coarsely touched than it ever had been since the days of the dear old doll, long buried in the garden" (ch. 9). A similar reaction marks Esther's first meeting with her mother, whom she has never known and who is still a mere stranger to her: "And, very strangely, there was something quickened within me, associated with the lonely days at my godmother's; yes, away even to the days when I had stood on tiptoe to dress myself at my little glass, after dressing my doll" (ch. 18).

Thus, underneath the narrative strand which moves toward Esther's social rootedness, there is the concern with the buried but stirring insistence of the original "wound" or "sin," which must be confronted to be cured or appeased. This confrontation happens, always at the level of implication, in stages. The first begins on the crucially important evening of Esther's contact with Jo, who will transmit the mysterious and highly contagious disease that originates from a rat scurrying from Captain Nemo's pauper grave in Tom-all-Alone's. At that moment, though Esther has not yet learned the identity of her mother—or even of her

19. The biblical Esther, a Jewish orphan and the ward of Mordecai, was chosen by the Babylonian King Ahasuerus to replace his wife Vashti, who had refused to appear dressed in nothing but the royal crown at a banquet held for the princes of the realm. Queen Esther was noted for a feminine diplomacy and manipulative respect for authority which allowed her to save her people from the extinction planned by Haman.

existence—she has the "undefinable impression" of "being something different from what I then was" (ch. 3). As Mark Spilka and Taylor Stoehr have suggested, this disease, never given a name in the novel, is on a symbolic level related to the unbridled sexuality of Esther's parents; and "smallpox" is indeed close enough to "pox" to assume a sexual connotation.[20]

In addition, smallpox, a disease which leaves pockmarks on the face, suggests the "wound" of castration of nonphallic origin. The imagery in which Esther describes the experience of her illness is suggestive of an archetypal and successful quest for identity—she recalls the sensation of crossing a dark lake and of laboring, like a worm, up colossal staircases; however, this confrontation with the uncanny taboo—the return of the repressed—does not lead to the blinding insight of a figure like Oedipus (though it strikes her with temporary blindness). Here is the *anagnorisis* when Esther looks at the pockmarks on her face:

> My hair had not been cut off. . . . It was long and thick. I let it down, and shook it out, and went up to the glass upon the dressing-table. There was a little muslin curtain drawn across it. I drew it back; and stood for a moment looking through such a veil of my own hair, that I could see nothing else. Then I put my hair aside, and looked at the reflection in the mirror. . . . I was very much changed—O very, very much. At first my face was so strange to me, that I think I should have put my hands before it and started back. . . . Very soon it became more familiar, and then I knew the extent of the alteration in it better than I had done at first. It was not like what I had expected; but I had expected nothing definite, and I dare say anything definite would have surprised me. [ch. 36]

In this revelation, in which Esther's social self finds her true self fearsomely *unfamiliar*, we recognize the same gesture of moving aside the hair to look at the face which marks the revelatory

20. M. Spilka, *Dickens and Kafka: A Mutual Interpretation* (Bloomington: Indiana University Press, 1963), p. 214; Stoehr, *Dickens*, pp. 143–44.

moment of Esther's later identification of and with her mother. Indeed, the frightening face surrounded by copious hair is an image of the Medusa's head, as Freud has told us, the visual representation of castrated female sexuality that turns the beholder into stone.[21] At one level, then, as a suggestive foreshadowing of the later event, this passage seems to imply Esther's acceptance of the biological truth of her origin without so much as touching the hem of Victorian respectability. However, in the evasiveness of the final phrases, refusing to accept loss or otherness in denying the existence of a previous expectation, her repression of the reality of her biological self is renewed.

Consequently, her illness results in an increased need to maintain the separateness of the split-off image of the doll rather than its integration. This shows itself in Esther's relationship to Ada Clare, who—like Charley, Esther's little maid—is a reincarnation of the long-buried doll. Charley's wide-eyed tininess suggests the childhood confidante, but Ada has its "beautiful complexion" and "rosy lips," and is, moreover, an idealized alter ego: contrary to the sexlessness indicated by Esther's nicknames (Mother Hubbard, Dame Durden, Mrs. Shipton), Ada represents feminine sexuality, as indicated by her betrothal to Richard; in contrast to Esther's sense of her own unworthiness, Ada seems bright, beautiful, good, and unblemished. No wonder that Esther seems to love Ada almost more than herself. When Ada marries Richard, Esther hopes to live with them; keeping "the keys of their house," she will be made "happy for ever and a day" (ch. 14). When her longing to reconstitute the triangle of family romance in this manner is not fulfilled, Esther is wild with grief. At night she steals to Ada's house and listens to the sounds within! During her illness, it is Ada's pure beauty which must be protected from the disease at all cost. Ada's perfection, the token that she has had no contact with the blight of natural female origin clinging to Esther, is "the light" in Esther's blindness. During her illness Esther seems to feel that without preserving

21. S. Freud, "Medusa's Head" (1922), *Standard Edition* (London: Hogarth, 1955), vol. 18.

this idealized version of herself uncontaminated and intact, she cannot continue to live: if Ada is allowed to look upon her marked face for only one moment, Esther will die.

Esther's continued fear of revealing her face to Ada marks her unchanged refusal to accept herself as her mother's daughter. From this point of view, it is highly significant that the chapter that has as its central event the relatively restrained recognition of the kinship between Esther and her mother should end in a climax of much greater emotional intensity with the reunion of Esther and Ada. Here we see Ada play the mother role, accepting Esther's face, "bathing it with tears and kisses, rocking [her] to and fro like a child, calling [her] by every tender name that she could think of" (ch. 36). Only after Esther has truly accepted the familiarity of her mother's "sin" will she change positions with Ada: whereas Esther has a romance and starts her own family, the widowed Ada moves back to Bleak House to take care of her guardian.

This moment of acceptance comes after another confrontation with the "sin" from which all corruption in *Bleak House* has started, after another archetypal descent, which, unlike Esther's illness, is a confrontation with real death. It is the death of Lady Dedlock, who has completed her own circuitous return to the reality of the past and lies dead at the grave of the man "who should have been her husband," in the spot from which all corruption in the world of this novel takes its origin. This final image of Tom-all-Alone's is the "primal scene" of the motivation of the narrative. From here the subversive threat of the leveling of hierarchical distinctions—of a breakdown of the walls of subjectivity that ensure the operative power of such concepts as race, class, sex, and age—has arisen, the threat of which the narrator asserts that "His Grace shall not be able to say Nay to the infamous alliance" (ch. 46). Esther's journey toward this heart of London's darkness, undertaken to "save" her mother from the final deed, leads her through a "labyrinth of streets," in between darkness and dawn, into a mental state between waking and dreaming in which the reality she had always known seems so changed that "great water-gates seemed to be opening and closing in my head, or in the air; and . . . the unreal things were more substantial than the real" (ch. 59). Directly preceding this, she has confessed that it seemed as if the "stained house-fronts put on human shapes and looked at" her; in the light of the house symbolism of the novel, this seems a hallucinatory realization that the stain of Tom-all-Alone's is also her own but cannot yet be admitted into consciousness. Thus, when she arrives at the entrance to this enclosed place—the curiously Victorian version of the *hortus conclusus*—she still cannot relate its otherness to herself:

> The gate was closed. Beyond it, was a burial-ground—a dreadful spot in which the night was very slowly stirring; but where I could dimly see . . . houses . . . on whose walls a thick humidity broke out like a disease. On the step at the gate, drenched in the fearful wet of such a place, which oozed and splashed down everywhere, I saw, with a cry of pity and horror, a woman lying—Jenny, the mother of the dead child. [ch. 59]

But this last phrase is not final; it is to be revised into the "dead mother of the living child." The truth about her own face will come home after a gesture we remember from Esther's illness: "I lifted the heavy head, put the long dank hair aside, and turned the face. And it was my mother, cold and dead" (ch. 59). At last, then, the unfortunate girl has owned her mother, has looked the evil of her birth in the face and accepted it as her own; from this moment on the taboo on her sexuality is lifted. Avoiding the mistakes of her mother, Esther does not marry the elderly Jarndyce, who calls her "my child," but confesses her hitherto unacknowledged attraction to Alan Woodcourt.

III

Considered in the framework of the internal logic of this fiction, Esther's confrontation with the otherness of her origin has been necessary in order to gain full acceptance of her own identity and thus bring the narrative to a satisfactory closure. But the scene is equally necessary in terms of the discursive level of the text. Lady Dedlock must die in order to cleanse and purify—to exorcise—the implications of Esther's recognition. *Bleak House* is as much the inspired page, the literary signifier, proclaiming the redemption of the loss of presence resulting from original sin through the steady exercise of Victorian virtue; it provides the "key" of duty and order, functioning like a fig leaf to shield Victorian eyes from actually seeing what they know is there. This curious strategy of concealment and simultaneous revelation is inevitable since fictional discourse, *exemplum* and sustenance of the cultural order, cannot move outside the bounds of logocentrism without imperiling the grounds of its own existence; the repression or exclusion of the heterogeneous lends connectedness and meaning to the fiction. A full recognition and acceptance of Lady Dedlock's otherness would have destroyed the hierarchical order in which the binary pair "Father-M(other)" is positioned in the *Scala Naturae*. Letting Lady Dedlock live, reconciling her with her husband and daughter, would have "opened the floodgates" and erased "the principle of cohesion" upon which the revisionary narrative strain depends, something we see happen in the works of Joyce.

Though Dickens has obvious problems controlling the vision he evokes, he eventually stems the threat of engulfment, not only by killing Lady Dedlock but also by revising the notion of "the Father" in a strategic diversionary move reminiscent of the replacement of the castrating primal (Mosaic) father of the Old Testament by the figure of Jesus in the New Testament—of Old Law by the New—allaying the threat of retribution by a reduction in authoritative power and an emphasis on charity or agape.

The "old fathers"—Lord Dedlock and the Lord High Chancellor are, as I noted earlier, the most prestigious examples—have proven "Krooks," negative forces, hoarding life and energy for self-serving purposes; though Lord Dedlock's love for his wife redeems him to a certain extent, he is shown to us first and primarily as the typical embodiment of a reactionary force aiming at maintaining the status quo of the old dispensation. The first "new father," Mr. Jarndyce, on the other hand, is notable for the generosity with which he fulfills out of love the duties of the Lord

High Chancellor and provides for the orphans of chancery. A spokesman for Dickens' views, he keeps himself consciously aloof from legal and political entanglements and tries to preserve a prelapsarian enclave of sweetness and light in his home. To Esther he soon becomes a "father" whose goodness seems of divine origin, and he remains a source of inspiration till the end of the story, when she writes that at the moment the "sun's rays descended . . . upon his bare head, I felt as if the brightness on him must be the brightness of the Angels" (ch. 64).

What is important with regard to Dickens' revisionary strategy, however, is that as a father-figure Jarndyce is reluctant to assume authority. He appears to need the love of his wards to such an extent that he condescends to eradicate the social and emotional differences which separate them—by proposing to marry Esther. This he does, appropriately enough—in the context of both his position as a *deus*-figure and the importance of "writing" in this novel—in a letter. As a literary figure, Mr. Jarndyce seems to derive from a familiar eighteenth-century type, the benevolent gentleman, as the critics have repeatedly pointed out. But if we compare him with Rousseau's M. de Wolmar in *La Nouvelle Héloise,* with which the plot of Bleak House has striking structural and thematic similarities, one cannot help noting how much more "romantic" Dickens' figure is. Jarndyce eventually renounces possession of his promised bride, Esther, and arranges for her marriage to the man she secretly loves. This version of the *senex-*, or, by extension, *deus*-figure seems to result from the need to accommodate the wishes and allay the fears of the "self" of the writer, who does not or cannot identify with the overtly patriarchal figures of power and veers toward imaginative empathy with the underdog. The fact that Esther's marriage and her little house are, in the final analysis, made to seem dependent on the providence of this "new" father—rather than on the hard-won insights of her own experience—amounts to a neutralization of Esther's heterogeneity by this revised (and obviously effective) version of the myth of paternal origin.

The high romantic replacement of the faded numinosity of the Lord High Chancellor by the "brightness of the Angels" radiating from Jarndyce tells us something about the place of this fiction in literary history; however, more significant as an indication of its specifically Victorian aspects (and here we finally verge back toward our starting point in Darwin's *Origin of Species*), is the substitution of detective Bucket for Tulkinghorn as the agency which penetrates the secret of Lady Dedlock's otherness and resolves the mystery of origin.

Of all the characters Dickens has created in *Bleak House*, Tulkinghorn is the most mysteriously evil and the most convincing. Perhaps it is because he is in effect the "king," the most powerful and the most traditionally masculine personality of Dickens' stage, that his presence haunts the reader as it does Lady Dedlock; or it may be because of his curious relationship to the feebleness of the Lord High Chancellor: that which indicated the latter's failure, his inability to inspire and shine, becomes, with an inversion, the very source of power for Tulkinghorn. In his black clothes—which, peculiarly enough, never shine but seem "mute, close, irresponsive to any glancing light" (ch. 2)—he is like a black hole in space, a burned-out star, sucking everything around him inside the radius of his hoarding power. In his insufficiently lit room everything is locked away in a perverse exaggeration of Esther's proud housekeeping, but here even the key is hoarded and kept out of sight in a peculiar inversion of the castration motif. Tulkinghorn has no emotional ties to other people, no passions to break the rigidity of his black armor; his only desire is the acquisition of knowledge and secrets and "the holding possession of such power as they give him, with no sharer or opponent in it" (ch. 36). In a world where the key, the symbol of patriarchal power, is lost or unintelligible, Tulkinghorn has set out to embody this key himself, to be "all in all." While the feminine figure of allegory hangs over his head like the sword of Damocles, he "cuts her dead" and ignores what her name implies—the inevitable presence of otherness, the curse of writing—spying and prying all the while to contain the threatening secret of Lady Dedlock, to "cut her dead" through the force of his presence.

As Joseph Fradin suggests, Tulkinghorn, like Krook, is "allegorically" self-destroyed by the repression of his own deeper emotions—that is, unrestraint and passion, embodied in Lady Dedlock's maid Hortense.[22] His place in Sir Leicester's confidence and in the pursuit of Lady Dedlock is taken by another servant of the law, detective Bucket, who is in a sense the hero of this novel. In contrast to Tulkinghorn, he dispels the darkness and fog of origin, leading Esther to the moment of revelation in the pauper graveyard. Similarly, Bucket's power, seemingly preternatural—he is omnipresent, he has attendants everywhere, he penetrates secrets, and he moves about with infallible aim—is not the hoarding power of the older man but is the power of youth, mobility, sympathy, and wit. If Tulkinghorn as representative of an outworn ideal of masculinity is almost a *dio boia,* Bucket is the incarnation of the optimistic vitality of a newer version, based on the nineteenth-century belief in the power of scientific investigation. Like Mephistopheles' shining and increasing key in *Faust II* (according to Carl Jung, a symbol of the phallus, like Tom Thumb and other "dactyls"),[23] Bucket's extended forefinger leads Esther down to the crucial place, the realm of the mother. It is Bucket's forcefulness which unlocks Esther's sexuality. And in making Esther's revelation dependent upon the agency of this detective, Dickens seems to be offering an additional replacement for the faded numinosity and effectiveness of the primal father(s) of this fiction, in the form of a newer hero and a more socially constructive use of power.

Dickens' strategy for containing the disruptive heterogeneity of the female, or of nature, through the replacement of the old father(s) by new fathers, is itself the revisionary movement we recognize from the family romance, lending an extra, literal edge to his well-known avowal in the preface of having "purposely dwelt upon the romantic side of *familiar things*" (my emphasis). Indeed, it would be foolish to blame Dickens for a lack of intellectual consistency, for revealing and repressing at the same time. Not only is *Bleak House* a fiction, aiming at a different kind of

22. Fradin, "Will and Society," pp. 103–04.

23. C. G. Jung, *Symbols of Transformation: An Analysis of the Prelude to a Case of Schizophrenia,* trans. R.F.C. Hull (New York: Harper, 1956), pp. 124 ff.

truth from that emerging in a work of philosophy, but the mind, as it expresses itself in language, cannot step outside the very play of polarities that make significance and communication possible. It would have been inconceivable to let *Bleak House* take the course of *Ulysses* or *Finnegan's Wake,* where Molly Bloom and Anna Livia Plurabelle flood the discursiveness of form, structure, and language with their otherness. Without Jarndyce's benevolence and Bucket's intervention, Esther's children could not have been born.

Moreover, if we compare Dickens' revisionary strategy with that of Darwin, this strategy proves suggestive of a general pattern for the age, not one limited to fiction. While Darwin writes a work of science, still, like the writer of narrative, he must cut and tie the strands of his argument to arrive at a convincing, meaningful conclusion. Rereading the last chapter of *The Origin of Species* one notes that the threat to human self-respect implied in an evolutionary notion of origin—that man is not created separately in God's image, or, even worse, that there is no definite moment of transcendental origin—is lessened by the author's implied suggestion that a revised interpretation of the biblical account might picture the creator as a prime mover impressing his laws upon matter, not as the anthropomorphic father shaping his children in clay.

IV

The polarities of father-mother, creator-matter, are intrinsic to human thought, whether fictional or scientific; it is not their mere presence or opposition but their internal relationship, the manner in which they inform a narrative strategy or a scientific argument, which is significant for the epistemological concerns of an age. Thus, this analysis of the symbolic structure of *Bleak House* need not lead us into the alley of critical self-involvement or tie us inextricably into a self-spun tropological net. On the contrary, if the analogy with the conceptual structure of the *Origin of Species* has a function, it is this: it may help us to gain a clearer vision of the historical development of the novel in relation to the ontological concerns of the age in which it takes its existence, and which it embodies in turn. In other words, I am contending that *Bleak House* as a fiction is not merely the personal nightmare of its author or a literary pacifier, superficially reflecting and removed from the strife of historical existence. I believe that as a work of serious and compassionate art it addresses itself in its peculiarly fictional form to a mid-nineteenth-century embodiment of an ineradicable human problem, and that consequently its narrative strategy assumes literary-historical significance. Further, as I shall try to show, it clarifies the transition from an earlier plot structure predominent in popular fiction (and Dickens' own earlier novels), the simple family romance, to that typically Victorian form, the detective story. Both share features of hidden origin and miraculous, sudden discovery.

Though *Bleak House* has many features of the older family romance, the moment which resolves the original blight, the discovery of the dead mother at the entrance to Tom-all-Alone's, is reached only after a deliberate, organized search, directed by a trained professional. Unlike the popular family romance, which assumes that identity is there merely waiting to be discovered, *Bleak House* is notable for its fairly early revelation of origin (in itself a reconstitution) and its lengthy process of bringing Lady Dedlock, the criminal, to what is in terms of Victorian narrative logic her justly deserved end. But this logic is Victorian not only because of the emphasis on the process of excommunication rather than mere discovery: the nature of what is communicated is of equal importance. Thus, in the light of psychoanalytic theories of the detective story, it is curiously appropriate that the moment at Tom-all-Alone's, while not a revelation of the crime of murder, should be both the revelation of a moment of pathetic death, and a displaced version of the primal scene. In her analysis of Poe's "The Murders in the Rue Morgue," Marie Bonaparte writes: "The unconscious source of our interest in narratives of this type lies, as Freud first led us to recognize, in the fact that the researches conducted by the detective reproduce, by displacement onto subjects of a quite different nature, our infantile investigations into matters of sex."[24] In other words, the detective story, displacing the primal scene onto a scene of violence, offers the reader an opportunity to allay his fear and curiosity without having to acknowledge it.

But what is "primal scene" but another term for the moment of biological origin? And if it is true that biological origin as a problem is characteristic of the Victorian age, can we not, in turn, explain the origin and popularity of the detective story as the fictional reflection of the deeper, unconscious concerns of the age? However, unconscious concern with origin can account for only one aspect of the mystery story, its fascination with violence. As a fiction privileging organized investigation, rational detection rather than accidental discovery, the detective novel is the fictional form of an epoch which has committed itself to a belief in the liberating efficacy of scientific research. As Hartman writes, "It explains the irrational . . . by the latest rational system."[25] The "whodunit" is the poor, or less prestigious, stepsister of a scientific treatise like the *Origin of Species,* and Darwin's injunction that we "possess no pedigrees or armorial bearings" [i.e., fixed origin], and "we have to *discover* and *trace* the many diverging lines of descent in our natural genealogies" (my emphasis), conforms to what the detective novel, in its characteristically displaced form, does.

Probably because of its experimental searching for an adequate

24. M. Bonaparte, "The Murders in Rue Morgue," *Psychoanalytic Quarterly* 4 (1935): 259–93, p. 292. The connection between detective story and "primal scene" was first brought to my attention by Geoffrey H. Hartman's "Literature High and Low: The Case of the Mystery Story," in *The Fate of Reading: And Other Essays* (Chicago: University of Chicago Press, 1975). Hartman speaks of "one definitively visualized scene to which everything else might be referred," a "scene of suffering" or a "to pathos" (p. 207). His argument also refers to the work of Charles Rycroft, "The Analysis of a Detective Story," in *Imagination and Reality: Psychoanalytical Essays 1951–61* (London: Hogarth, 1968), and of Geraldine Pedersen-Krag, "Detective Stories and the Primal Scene," *Psychoanalytic Quarterly* 18 (1949): 207–14. I have relied on all these works in reaching my conclusions.

25. Hartman, "Literature High and Low," p. 209.

form *Bleak House* is both more primitive and less displaced than the more sophisticated work of Dickens' friend Wilkie Collins and his acquaintance Poe, though the indebtedness to "The Purloined Letter" (1845) seems especially great.[26] Thus, what Hartman calls the "scene of suffering" is displaced by a scene of recognition both more clearly sexual and more ambivalent than the central event in the crime mystery. I say more ambivalent, because in the detective novel the "parent for whom the reader (the child) has negative oedipal feelings" is represented as the pitiful victim, whereas Lady Dedlock, the dead mother, is both victim and criminal at once.[27] *Bleak House* shows us in the moment at Tom-all-Alone's a "whodunit" off guard as a "Hawdon-it," and this lesser depth of its "buried life" seems to provide unique insight into the generic moment of transformation from (family) romance into detective novel.

With this realization we have arrived at a better position from which to judge the validity of the initial assumption of this essay—that Dickens' concern with orphanhood in *Bleak House* and other writings, and the revisionary tactics with which he excommuni-

26. Thus we know from the very beginning who the criminal is: a woman whose prominent social position places her in the public eye. Moreover, the "crime" relates to a piece of writing, a personal letter, suggesting illicit personal relations. Apart from the gusty autumn weather of the setting, the analogy extends to the similarity in character of Tulkinghorn and Mr. D——, who hoard the secret, and their replacement in the plot by the detectives Bucket and Dupin. An interesting psychoanalytic interpretation of Poe's story, which confirms by analogy this reading of *Bleak House,* is in J. Lacan, "The Seminar on *The Purloined Letter,*" trans. J. Mehlman, *French Freud, Yale French Studies* 48 (1972). Lacan's interpretation has been criticized by Jacques Derrida in "Le Facteur de la Verité," *Poetique* 21 (1975): 96–147. For an exposition of Lacan's analysis, see S. Felman, "On Reading Poetry: Reflections on the Limits and Possibilities of Psychoanalytic Approaches," in J. H. Smith, ed., *The Literary Freud: Mechanisms of Defense and the Poetic Will,* vol. 4 of *Psychiatry and the Humanities* (New Haven: Yale University Press, 1980).

Dickens had met Poe in Philadelphia during his American tour of 1842, and had promised to find an English publisher for *Tales of the Grotesque and Arabesque.* Though publication of "The Purloined Letter" postdates their meeting, it seems unlikely that Dickens, who had kept in touch with Poe, would not have read this *Tale.*

27. Pedersen-Krag, "Detective Stories," p. 209.

cates the threat of otherness from the surface level of his novel, should not be seen as merely reflecting a personal psychological need or the artistic credo that "in all familiar things, even in those which are repellent on the surface, there is Romance enough, if we will find it out."[28] Dickens, as the strategist of his narrative, is an analogue of the energetic detective Bucket, searching and finding out with his pen—guided by his pointed forefinger—the (dis)closure of Esther's illegitimate origin;[29] and just as Bucket's mysterious powers dissolve the anxiety of his world, Dickens' narrative magic wipes the cobwebs of doubt from the Victorian sky, giving his audience on an unconscious level what it needs to pull through, *the reassuring message of the familiar myth.*

28. From "A Preliminary Word," in the first number of *Household Words,* 30 March 1850, when Dickens was writing *David Copperfield.*

29. Dickens had originally pictured his authorial persona for *Household Words* as a "certain SHADOW, which may go into any place, by sunlight, moonlight, starlight . . . and be supposed to be cognizant of everything." This reminds one rather suggestively of Bucket's omnipresent omniscience. See E. Johnson, *Charles Dickens: His Tragedy and Triumph* (New York: Viking Press, 1952; rev. ed. 1977), pp. 356 ff.

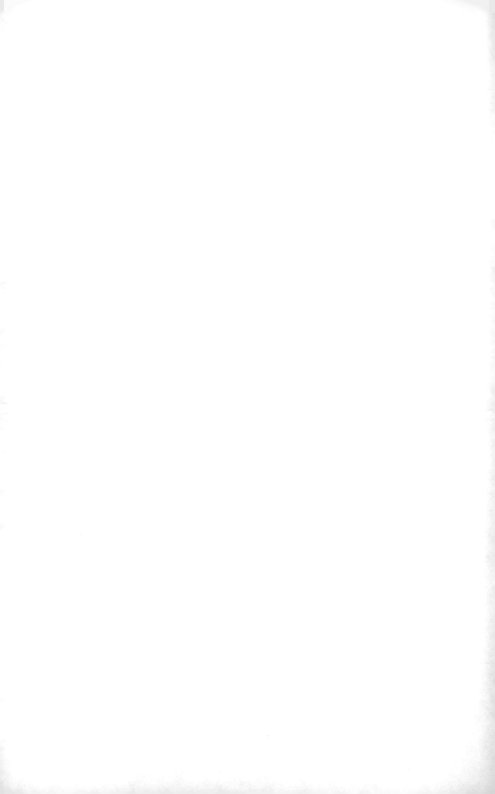

Epilogue:

Lacan and the Subject of American Psychoanalysis

Joseph H. Smith

The reader previously unacquainted with Jacques Lacan's work may benefit by a brief review of several potential stumbling blocks variously addressed in the preceding chapters. For the psychoanalyst, especially the American psychoanalyst, these would center mainly on Lacan's concept of the ego, the virtual usurpation of the economic point of view by a linguistic point of view, and, within the latter, an uncertain concept or sense of reference. I shall outline these three areas and suggest at least a few possible points of consensus between Lacan's thought and ego psychology.

In Lacan's reading of Freud, the ego emerges solely in its defensive aspect. I would therefore suggest that Lacan be studied with an eye for a profound and new insight into the possibilities of defensive ego functioning. But beyond that, at some point, one must attend the ambiguity inherent in the concept of defense itself.

The psychoanalytic concept of defense depends upon the assumption of a truth of outer and inner worlds which defense distorts. Where there is no warrant for such an assumption the concept of defense is baseless, even though it still may be indispensable. There would be, for instance, no warrant for that assumption in the individual's coming into being as an individual. There we can only assume an absence of differentiated outer and inner worlds.[1] The question is the role of defense in their being constituted. But defense (or protodefense) at such a point is revealed as a paradox—as harboring opposite and contradictory meanings in the sense that defensive action negatively acknowledges and thereby is a first step in constituting that which it defends against.

Take the identity of perception—the presumed early hallucination of the breast (however represented) by the hungry infant. Can we say this is a defense against the absence of the mother? Why not?—provided we have in mind that at this stage there is no mother or any subject of the defending and that it is at once defense against the absence of the object and also a first sketch of both object and subject, a first step in the constitution of object and subject and in that order. The identity of perception would not be just a wrong alley that must be forsaken for the identity of thought. It *is* that, but it is also the access *to* thought, understood as beginning with an image of the object that is the goal of thought and action.

This same constituting function would also hold for Lacan's mirror stage—the fascination, even captivation, of the eight-month-old by his image in a mirror or by some semblance of wholeness or integrity reflected to him as more than he is in the mother's caretaking—and the whole "series of alienating identifi-

1. The definite evidence of astonishing competencies in the neonate brought to light by the sophisticated methods of current infant observation would be taken by many as rendering immediately obsolete not only Lacanian but also many of Freud's and Piaget's inferences and assumptions regarding early psychic development. Infants in the very first weeks show a remarkable "pre-wired" capacity to "differentiate" the mother from others (Stern, 1983). I have outlined elsewhere (Smith, 1983), however, reasons for believing that such early competence is a different phenomenon than the differentiations the infant becomes capable of at eight months or those marked by the advent of language. It is a matter of awareness of awareness (Rapaport, 1957, p. 329). The difference between knowing something and knowing that one knows it is the difference between being there as a subject and not yet being there. How subjecthood in this sense is gradually achieved through infancy and early childhood may also become subjects for infant research. Until the findings of that research are established, Freud's inferences regarding early development based on regressive phenomena, rough though they be, are still pertinent.

cations" by which the ego, for Lacan, is "constituted in its nucleus" (*Écrits*, p. 128). In reference to Lacan's Schéma R, Green writes herein that the "(*a*), in its relation to *a'* (which will be closely related to the future i(*a*), i.e., the mirror image) can be understood as an *element of ineluctable mediation* uniting the subject with the Other" (p. 64). He further writes:

> If *A* [*Autre*—Other with a capital O], to attain its full significance, requires the support of the *Name-of-the-Father* . . . it passes along the maternal route and becomes effective only when the break between the subject and the maternal object separates irremediably the two entities. . . . Thus, the *objet (a)* . . . attains the status of the object of desire. . . .
>
> The location of this object in the field of the Other allows us, therefore, to conceive of the function of mediation that such an object plays out. [pp. 167–68]

This is to say that even within Lacan's own view, ego development is a necessary step toward and foothold for assuming one's subjectivity, even though psychoanalysis, according to Lacan, ought to be a method for dissolution of the ego by virtue of which the patient is enabled to more nearly approach the being of the I, the true subject.

For Lacan the ego is thus the false self that he wrongly assumed American ego psychology took to be the center of the true self. But in ego psychology it is not assumed that ego as agency is the subject. The subject—the "I" that is constructed and assumed during development—is the self. But this is not the self of Kohut or a self-psychology, and certainly not merely the integrate of self-representations as in Kernberg (1975, pp. 315–16). In ego psychology the self is marked out, not thematized. Notwithstanding the effort by Hartmann (1950, pp. 84–85) and others, it is still without conceptual status. It does not enter as a concept in the theory of ego psychology and psychoanalytic intervention. In a sense, just as fixations and conflicts are elucidated in order to enhance the power of choice, the assumption of the self is left to the patient.

I now turn to the usurpation of the economic point of view by the linguistic. The whole debate on whether or how the unconscious is structured like a language hinges on the question of psychic energy. It is central in Ricoeur's critique and is explicitly or implicitly at issue in every chapter of this book. For various reasons—among them the frequent confusion of the concepts of psychic energy and of affect, to which I shall return—it is a subject that calls for explicit comment here.

The thing to bear in mind about psychic energy is that it *is* psychic. To hold to such a concept is not to biologize psychology, as Woody herein, for instance, seems to believe. In David Rapaport's words:

> We must keep in mind that in dealing with instinctual drives and the energy they expend in their work, we are not speaking about the muscular or other physiological energy expended . . . but rather about the psychological energy expended in the initiation, regulation and termination of behaviour—the physiological, biochemical, biophysical, or neurophysiological substrate of which we know, so far, nothing. [1960, p. 874]

The more general statement of the point by Ricoeur is as follows:

> Dynamic concepts are applicable to several regions without belonging to any. In the "region" of things or in the "region" of consciousness there are many . . . concepts [that] . . . overlap all "regions," as the terms object, property, relation, plurality, etc. Phenomenology of consciousness requires dynamics, just as it requires other concepts of "formal ontology." It is even possible to construct a purely psychological dynamics without reference to physics or even psychology. It was to avoid the sliding of psychological dynamics (with its concepts of force, tension, release, etc.) into a physical interpretation that we have held the description of willing as force in suspension until now and that we have considered it as thought, that is as practical, a-dynamic intention. Now we must not forget that voluntary and involuntary *forces* are also

the forces which evoke or actualize a *meaning*. [1950, pp. 224–25]²

It is too often assumed that instinctual drives in Freud are clearly phenomena of one region, the somatic, represented in another region, the psyche, by ideation and affect.

But Freud wrote:

> If now we apply ourselves to considering mental life from a *biological* point of view, an "instinct" appears to us as a concept on the frontier between the mental and the somatic, as the psychical representative of the stimuli originating from within the organism and reaching the mind, as a measure of the demand made upon the mind for work in consequence of its connection with the body. [1915, pp. 121–22]

Rapaport, the most rigorously systematic of American ego psychologists, commented:

> Here in the term "psychical representative," the term "representative" is not the same as in the term "drive representation" . . . [i.e.,] affects and ideas. That the instinct here is "psychical representative" means simply that we can't talk about it in terms of physiology. . . . That doesn't mean that one can't use physiological analogies; that doesn't mean that one cannot bring in patterns of thought derived from physiology. But the theory is a psychological theory. . . . The instinct *is* the mental representation . . . the mental representative, as we should put it, of . . . organic stimuli. [1959, pp. 270–71]

Loewald's comment on the same passage bears quoting at length:

> Instinct, understood as a psychical representative (*Repräsentant*), is not a stimulus impinging on the psychic apparatus but is a force within or of the psychic apparatus; a force

---

2. See also similar statements by Kurt Lewin in Rapaport (1960, pp. 873–74) and by Loewald (1971, pp. 100–01).

which represents stimuli originating in the body in a different, i.e., psychical, form. . . . We must distinguish between
psychic representative (*Repräsentant* and *Repräsentanz*) and
representation in the sense of idea (*Vorstellung*). The meaning of representation, as used in the word representative, is
wider than that of representation as idea. Psychical representation in the wider sense includes, for instance, such non-
ideational phenomena as affects and, of course, as we have
seen, instincts. . . . Mental or psychical representatives are
hierarchically structured in such a way that representatives
of a lower order can be rerepresented—not *necessarily* in the
form of ideas—on higher mental levels. . . .

Instincts then, considered from a so-called biological point
of view, are mental stimuli. The system in which physiological stimuli are represented as instincts is capable of representing. What may be said to be stimulated by physiological,
organic stimuli (and, we may assume, by other kinds of physical stimuli as well) is this faculty of representing, an activity
which is then seen as inherent in the mind and not brought to
it from the organismic needs. . . . My accent is not on the fact
that instincts are mental representatives of organismic stimuli, but on the fact that they are mental representatives.
[1971, pp. 107–09]

I submit that the concepts of psychic energy and of instinct or
instinctual drive in Rapaport and Loewald (together with those of
Schafer, discussed below) are at least closer to Lacan's concept of
desire (and thus more compatible with the position that the unconscious is structured like a language) than to the concepts of
energy and instinct as biological phenomena that French writers
still take as holding sway in the United States. I also submit that
the Lacanian notion of a dynamics of desire is not so far removed
as he thought from the concepts of force and energy for which he
derided his American colleagues. It is not a matter of Lacanian
thought *needing* a concept of energy, as Ricoeur, Kristeva, and
Vergote argue; Lacan *had* a concept of energy, unacknowledged
but embedded in his dynamics (he would have said in his dialec-

JOSEPH H. SMITH

tics) of desire. Desire is impelling, directional, i.e., a force, and
"like all force concepts [of any region] it involves a concept of
energy" (Rapaport, 1960, p. 874; see also Schafer, 1968, p. 43).
The question is whether or in what way the energy concept there
needs to be acknowledged.

There is now no doubt that for a long period in psychoanalysis
the economic point of view was pressed into carrying far more
than its share of explanatory value. In the process the energy
concept was reified—not only in those instances where it was
taken literally as being physical energy, but also where it was
taken on psychological ground as an entity that could of itself
account for its referents. The referents of psychic energy (or
cathexis or economics) "are the signs of strength, influence, or
importance of certain motives" (Schafer, 1968, p. 43). When we
attempt to explain such strength, influence, or importance by
saying, for instance, that there is a large quotient of energy deployed, we are involved in pseudoexplanation—in fact, patent
tautology. The strength of the motive has to be explained on
other grounds and thus the importance and interdependence of
the five metapsychological points of view (Rapaport and Gill,
1959).

In his second theory of anxiety Freud was already backing away
(overcompensating, in fact, by backing away a bit too far) from
reliance on economic explanation: "Whereas I formerly believed
that anxiety invariably arose automatically by an economic process, my present conception of anxiety as a signal given by the ego
in order to affect the pleasure-unpleasure agency does away with
the necessity of considering the economic factor" (1926, p. 140).

It is my assumption that both ego psychology and Lacanian
theory had their major impetus as moves to counter economic
pseudoexplanation. It was for this reason, I believe, that Lacan
did not elaborate a dynamic or economic (energic) point of view
but left them implicit in desire.[3] Ego psychology, on the other

3. "Desire" is a force and thus both dynamic and economic. The dynamic refers
to the directional aspect or the aim of a force; the economic to the energic aspect
(Schafer, 1968, p. 43).

hand, while attempting to counter the economic by emphasizing the structural and adaptive (without, of course, the conformist implications that Lacan attributed to it) points of view, nevertheless allowed a radically wrong elaboration of the energy concepts to evolve in the midst of the new emphasis. What was wrong was the postulation of three different kinds of psychic enery (libidinal, aggressive, and neutral or neutralized) together with following Freud in a reified notion of the fusion and defusion of instincts. The former attributes quality or direction to a quantitative concept, thus blurring the distinction from the aim aspect of force. This could foster a bypassing of the task of understanding the set of conditions under which a libidinal or aggressive or neutral aim comes into being together with the set of conditions that determine the relative strength or weakness of such aims. The idea of fusion and defusion treats energy virtually as substance.

Regarding fusion and defusion, Ricoeur wrote:

> Fusion and defusion are simply the correlates, in energy language, of phenomena discovered by the work of interpretation when it focuses on the area of the instinctual representatives. [1970, p. 297]

Similarly, Schafer (1968, p. 214) defines fusion and defusion in terms of the compatibility or synthesis (or the lack thereof) of specific libidinal and aggressive aims.

In a comparable view of instinctual drives generally, Loewald wrote:

> Anything that we can call instinctual drives, as psychic forces, arise and are being organized first within the matrix of the mother-child unitary psychic field. . . . Instincts, in other words, are to be seen as relational phenomena from the beginning and not as autochthonous forces seeking discharge . . . understood as some kind of emptying of energy potential, in a closed system or out of it. [1972, p. 242]

The particular conflict of interpretations here discussed has often been taken as presenting only a black-or-white choice: biological energy as in ego psychology or no energy as in Lacan. I have shown above how the conflict could reach this degree of sharpness only by virtue of a careless or tendentious reading of both texts. A careful reading once again brings into view an area of compatibility ordinarily unrecognized by both Lacanians and ego psychologists. Both have an energy concept. In Lacan it is understated. The overstatement (and misstatement) of Hartmannian ego psychology has been corrected, I believe, by the formulations of Rapaport, Loewald, and Schafer cited.[4]

Before I leave the topic of psychic energy, a word can be added regarding the uncertain usage of the term *affect*. In Freud's first theory affect and energy were equated as "a quota of affect or sum of excitation—which possesses all the characteristics of a quantity" (1894, p. 60). This "affect" in Freud's theory of the instinctual drives became the energy—the cathexis—of the instinctual drives (Rapaport, 1960, p. 874). Subsequently, affect was distinguished from drive cathexis (Rapaport, 1953) and seen as one means of drive representation. Finally, in *Inhibitions, Symptoms and Anxiety* (1926), affect was conceptualized as conscious ego response with an emphasis on its signal function (Smith, 1970).

To my knowledge Ricoeur's clear statement above showing that psychological energy need not be taken as neurophysiological energy is not matched in his writing by a clear conceptual differentiation of energy and affect. This conceptual blurring seems to pervade the French psychoanalytic literature. When Vergote, Kristeva, and Green, for instance, question Lacan's inattention to affect, it is not always certain in which sense they are using the term. Often, just as in Ricoeur, "affect" comports the concept of energy. Thus Vergote writes of "affective energy" (p. 219), and Kristeva writes of "affect" (meaning, I think, what English-speaking analysts would call "instinctual drive") as that

4. The corrections by Rapaport, Loewald, and Schafer from the pole of ego psychology seem to go toward meeting the corrections regarding affect/energy by Kristeva, Vergote, and Green that come in the opposite direction from the pole of Lacanian theory. Since each group has arrived at these directions not in response to but independently of the other, their meeting would seem to bespeak a confirmation above and beyond the ordinary.

which introduces heterogeneity into the discursive order (p. 34); elsewhere she lists "libido, desire, instinctual drive, affect" (p. 40) as virtual synonyms.

I assume that a major significance of Green's essay for French psychoanalysts is that it does differentiate affect and energy. In the view of affects as secondary signifiers, he approaches in many ways the theory of affect outlined by Rapaport (1967). Green's formulation, of course, arises from Lacanian theory and, like the Kristeva and Vergote chapters, goes toward correcting the inattention to affect in Lacan. However, unlike them, he does in the process of locating affect within the theory differentiate it from psychic energy.

The final area to be outlined—one that I can barely touch upon—is the place of language in Lacan's thought, together with his concept (or lack thereof) of reference.

Of his three orders, the Real, the Imaginary, and the Symbolic, the Real is at farthest remove. We and our world are constituted by language. The Real, the thing in itself, remains, as such, unknowable. Needs, for instance, are real, but we come to know them only as they are represented as desire, at first in the image—a form of signification and thus a part of language in the broad sense—and later in the word. The world of images, of fantasy, of wish fulfillment, is the Imaginary order. It is the dominant order of the pre-oedipal period notwithstanding the beginning of speech during that era. The definitive passage to the Symbolic order, the world of language, law, and institutions, is by way of the oedipal crisis. The passage does not do away with the Imaginary. On the contrary, it is in the light of the Symbolic order that the Imaginary is situated *as* Imaginary. Analysis, in the Lacanian view, addresses failures in the enactment of this passage and overcomes them through the transference/countertransference reenactment. For Lacan, in summary, man is language. Our only access to the Real is via language, and the Imaginary and the Symbolic are themselves linguistic orders.

Let us follow briefly what might be seen as the flowering of Freud's linguistic bent in the thought of Lacan on the signifier, on his assertion that the unconscious is structured like a language, and on his resistance to the referential function of language. The foregoing discussion provides the basis for suggesting that for this flowering to prove fruitful it must be rejoined with the concepts of instinct, energy, and reference that are seemingly, at least at the surface level, bypassed in Lacan's move.

Instinct or instinctual drive may be a borderline concept, but, as the above citations demonstrate, it is taken by Rapaport and Loewald to be on the psychological side of the border. Physiological disequilibrium evokes a psychological disequilibrium as protorepresentation of the former. At a second level this psychological disequilibrium as instinct or instinctual drive is represented in the form of ideation and affect. As I have shown, both Rapaport (1957, pp. 270–71; 1959, p. 350) and Loewald (1980, pp. 117–19, 126, 129, 132, 135, 208, 326), though in different terminology, discuss these two levels of representation. The function of ideation and affect refers proximally to the prior level of protorepresentation, the latter a representative of physiological processes and a first level of coming into and belonging to the world as a subject. If the unconscious is structured like a language, this must refer to the second level of representation. Attention to both levels, however, should allow not only for the dominant place given to language in Lacan's thought but also for instinct and reference.

The foremost exponent of rejoining the economic and the linguistic has been Ricoeur (1970). We can also turn to him for a hint of at least one way in which reference might be reinstated. But let us first follow Lacan's drift away from energy and reference.

In *Écrits* (1977) Lacan wrote that it is illusion to believe "that the signifier answers to the function of representing the signified, or better, that the signifier has to answer for its existence in the name of any signification whatever" (p. 150). Muller and Richardson (1979) paraphrase or interpret: "It is illusion to think that the signifier serves to represent the signified" (p. 361). First of all, it should be noted that the meaning of "signified" in Lacan has glided appreciatively away from the tie to "signifier" in its Saussurean source. For Saussure "the linguistic sign unites not a thing and a name, but a concept and a sound image. . . . [It] is . . . a two-sided psychological entity . . . intimately united, and each recalls the other" (1966, p. 66). The concept was the signified and the sound-image the signifier. The signified constitutes the meaning of a particular signifier. But let us depart from Saussure and stay with what I take to be Lacan's usage. Perhaps the subject matter he addressed required modification and elaboration of the signifier/signified concepts. He is, after all, deploying them, now in the form of what he calls an algorithm, to elucidate transference, repression, metaphor, metonymy, desire, empty speech, full speech—in a word, everything.

One reason for seeing as illusion that the signifier serves to represent the signified is that the signifier is a ring "of a necklace that is a ring in another necklace made of rings" (1977, p. 153), in such fashion that the meaning of the signifier constituted by its connection in the chain overrides its capacity for arbitrary referential meaning. Language, that is, is not limited to a noun function of merely naming. It is a system in which the meaning of every signifier depends on its difference from every other signifier. Lacan phrased it in the extreme: "Only the correlations between signifier and signifier provide the standard for all research into signification" (p. 153).

A signifier can be replaced by another signifer and then, repressed, occupy the rank of the signified. It is the signified but as such is a latent or unconscious signifier. Notice how everything linguistic, everything semiotic, is coming to be taken as signifier—either conscious or unconscious—and the nature of the signified becomes, at least in my reading, elusive.

For some of us it may help to insert here a more Freudian phrasing of how repression "perpetuates the interval onto which another chain of signifiers can be grafted" (Muller and Richardson, 1979, p. 373). If desire leads toward danger, anxiety is evoked and the signifier of the desire is repressed. But desire does not rest and finds another signifier or successively a whole chain of signifiers—is this the gliding of the signified under the signifier?—all of which may be also inadmissible to consciousness until one or a series of signifiers is found that express the desire in such fashion as not to evoke the prospect of danger. That signifier is the metaphor replacing the original repressed signifier. The repressed signifier is now unconsciously grafted onto the whole chain of signifiers that could not be admitted to consciousness. All of these latent signifiers now are at the rank of the signified in relation to the newly implanted signifier.

Where, at such a point, is the truth of the subject? Are we to think that it is covered over by repression, or has a new truth embodied in the covering signifier been achieved?

I would say that a new truth has been attained but that it remains muted and fettered, the new signifier as much captive to the old as the old is subject to the new, so long as repression obtains—so long, that is, as the newly implanted signifier is deployed primarily for defensive purposes. The new truth is set free, paradoxically, to the extent that its bondage to the old is acknowledged. Only with the assumption of its history, its connection and derivation from the old and the repressed, can the new signifier function as the metaphor through which a new truth of the subject is established.

"The agency of the letter in the unconscious of reason since Freud" (Lacan, 1977, pp. 146–78) was to justify Lacan's thesis that the unconscious is structured like a language, a phrasing that he will clarify only to the point of saying we should take it literally, i.e., it is not a simile. But what is it to say that it is structured like a language and what specifically beyond its not being simile is it to take that literally? Does he mean structured *like* a language, and if so, how like a language? Does he mean the unconscious is *in and of* language—"belongs to the domain of language" (Vergote, p. 196)? Does he mean, that is, structured *by* language or so structured as to *be* a language? Lévi-Strauss (1967, p. 47), after all, did not conclude that the kinship system is like a language but that it "is a language." I hear something of that in Lacan's statement that "like a language" should be taken literally. Muller, Richardson, Casey and Woody, and Leavy herein seem to do some such thing, whether out of conviction or an effort at this stage to introduce and explain Lacanian theory rather than to offer a critique. It is a position questioned by Kristeva and Vergote. It is a position from

which Green departs by raising the question of Lacan's inattention to affect and then rejoins (but not without changing that
which he rejoins) by defining affect as a "secondary signifier."

Kristeva maintains that any attempt to liken the Freudian or
even Lacanian problematic to linguistic models can never be
more than an artifice that ignores the radical difference between
the two fields. Language, she believes, should be considered as a
"*process of signifiance*' in which the heterogeneity of two separate
modes should be distinguished: the *semiotic*, emanating from instinctual drives and primary processes; and the *symbolic*, assimila-
ble to secondary processes" (p. 34).

In the final section of her essay she stresses that the analytic
listening "not only to the content but also to the *dynamic of the sign*"
leads to "*infra-semantic*" insights, and these are the ultimate
guides for verbal intervention. Providing that intervention in the
form of "constructive" interpretation is not just to provide a
"holding pattern"—a view that could foster the idea of the cure as
a "reduction of the subject to the egoic or imaginary dynamic of
the mother-child relation"—but to offer instead interpretations
as "the *solder* [*soudure*] of the signifying function in its logical,
syntactical dimension" (pp. 48, 46) with the aim of repairing symbolic deficiencies consequent to a prior absence of the paternal
function.[5]

Lacan's seeming resistance to the referential dimension of language underlies both his concept of the signifier and his assumption that the unconscious is structured like a language. But is it
possible that Lacan downplays a "naming" or "descriptive" referential function in such fashion as to allow a more originary referential function to come into view? If so, his overall work would be
more compatible with Ricoeur's thought than might be suspected
at first glance.

In his critique of Lacan's (and Edelson's 1975) linguistic refor-

5. It is often said that Freud neglected the pre-oedipal mother-child relationship. Indeed, the advances in psychoanalysis over the past forty years have largely
come in a deeper understanding of that era. However, Kristeva here illustrates
one way in which Lacanian practice is a return to Freud in underscoring the
paternal function of analytic intervention.

mulation of psychoanalytic theory, Ricoeur maintains "that the universe of discourse appropriate to the analytic experience is not that of language but that of the image" (1978, p. 293). Of course, that would have given no pause to Lacan, who would have simply taken the image as a signifier within the structure of language in a broad sense. But Ricoeur argues that "it is mistaken to believe that everything semiotic is linguistic" (p. 311). His emphasis on the image, the imagination, and fantasy in general is based on a belief that "the articulation of the economic and the semiotic aspects of psychoanalysis [are thereby made] intelligible, whereas a purely linguistic theory seems to make them almost incomprehensible" (p. 322).

His presupposition is "not that everything is language, it is rather that it is always within a language that . . . experience is articulated" (1979, p. 216) and no mode of language is without referential function.

The extreme instance is poetry:

If some have held the poetic function of discourse to exclude its referential function, this was because, at first, the poem (. . . understood in a wide sense that includes narrative fiction, lyricism, and the essay) suspends a first-order referential function, whether it is a question of direct reference to familiar objects of perception or of indirect reference to physical entities that science reconstructs as underlying the former objects. In this sense, it is true that poetry is a suspension of the descriptive function. It does not add to our knowledge of objects. But this suspension is the wholly negative condition for the liberation of a more originary referential function, which may be called second-order only because discourse that has a descriptive function has usurped the first rank in daily life, assisted, in this respect, by science. Poetic discourse is also about the world, but not about the manipulable objects of our everyday environment. It refers to our many ways of belonging to the world before we oppose ourselves to things understood as "objects" that stand before a "subject." If we have become blind to these modalities of

rootedness and *belonging-to* (*appartenance*) that precede the relation of a subject to objects, it is because we have, in an
uncritical way, ratified a certain concept of truth, defined by
adequation to real objects and submitted to a criterion of
empirical verification and falsification. Poetic discourse precisely calls into question these uncritical concepts of adequation and verification. In so doing, it calls into question the
reduction of the referential function to descriptive discourse
and opens the field of a non-descriptive reference to the
world. [1979, p. 218; for a more extended and technical
treatment of the topic see Ricoeur, 1977, pp. 219–56]

Notwithstanding the lack of specific explication, Lacan's work,
in my reading, does open the field of a nondescriptive reference
to the world and a nondescriptive reference to the subject.

Is it a "return to Freud"? Is there in Freud that which Harold
Bloom (1978) reads as a catastrophic theory of development that
has been covered over in the history of psychoanalysis, in America and elsewhere? Does our current all-too-familiar picture of
Freud cover the uncanny force of a much less comforting figure,
as Sam Weber (1982, p. xvii) believes? Is our current self-psychology a vain attempt toward descriptive reference of a reified self, a
self fixed and tamed in order to be a proper object of descriptive
reference? If the subject is not that kind of object is it *scientific* to so
take it?

If we take Lacan's rejection of instinct and reference as a move
against reification of concepts and as a means of barring inap-
propriately descriptive reference, his linguistic reformulation of
the field does return us to a more unsettling Freud—a Freud who
would face American ego psychology with the question of what it
is to approach and repeatedly reapproach the assumption of
one's subjecthood, only to arrive at a symbolically structured acceptance that the center of one's being is decentered, other, never
fully present, never fixed. It is a question that pervades the text of
Lacan and also the expositions of his thought gathered in this
volume.

REFERENCES

Bloom, H. "Freud and the Poetic Sublime." *Antaeus* 30/31 (1978): 355–76.

Edelson, M. *Language and Interpretation in Psychoanalysis.* New Haven: Yale University Press, 1975.

Freud, S. *Standard Edition of the Complete Psychological Works.* London: Hogarth, 1953–74.
   "The Neuro-psychoses of Defence" (1894), vol. 3.
   "Instincts and Their Vicissitudes" (1915), vol. 14.
   Inhibitions, Symptoms and Anxiety (1926), vol. 20.

Hartmann, H. "Comments on the Psychoanalytic Theory of the Ego." *Psychoanalytic Study of the Child* 5 (1950): 74–96.

Kernberg, O. *Borderline Conditions and Pathological Narcissism.* New York: Jason Aronson, 1975.

Lacan, J. *Écrits: A Selection.* Translated by A. Sheridan. New York: Norton, 1977.

Lévi-Strauss, C. *Structural Anthropology.* Garden City, N.Y.: Anchor, 1967.

Loewald, H. "On Motivation and Instinct Theory." *The Psychoanalytic Study of the Child* 26 (1971): 91–128.

———. "Freud's Conception of the Negative Therapeutic Reaction, with Comments on Instinct Theory." *Journal of the American Psychoanalytic Association* 20 (1972): 235–45.

———. *Papers on Psychoanalysis.* New Haven: Yale University Press, 1980.

Muller, J., and Richardson, W. *Toward Reading Lacan: Pages for a Workbook,* ch. 5, "The Agency of the Letter in the Unconscious or Reason Since Freud." *Psychoanalysis and Contemporary Thought* 2 (1979): 345–75.

Rapaport, D. "On the Psychoanalytic Theory of Affects" (1953). In *The Collected Papers of David Rapaport.* Edited by M. Gill. New York: Basic Books, 1967.

———. *Seminars on Elementary Metapsychology.* Edited by S. C. Miller. Stockbridge, Mass.: Austen Riggs Center, 1957 and 1959 (mimeographed).

———. "On the Psychoanalytic Theory of Motivation" (1960). In *The Collected Papers of David Rapaport.* Edited by M. Gill. New York: Basic Books, 1967.

Rapaport, D., and Gill, M. "The Points of View and Assumptions of

Metapsychology" (1959). In *The Collected Papers of David Rapaport*. Edited by M. Gill. New York: Basic Books, 1967.

Ricoeur, P. *Freedom and Nature: The Volumtary and the Involuntary* (1950). Translated and with an introduction by E. Kohak. Evanston, Ill.: Northwestern University Press, 1966.

————. *Freud and Philosophy*. New Haven: Yale University Press, 1970.

————. *The Rule of Metaphor*. Translated by R. Czerny. Toronto: University of Toronto Press, 1977.

————. "Image and Language in Psychoanalysis." In J. H. Smith, ed., *Psychoanalysis and Language*, vol. 3 of *Psychiatry and the Humanities*. New Haven: Yale University Press, 1978.

————. "Naming God." *Union Seminary Quarterly Review* 34, no. 4 (1979): 215–27.

Saussure, F. de. *Course in General Linguistics*. Edited by C. Bally and A. Sechehaye. Translated by W. Baskin. New York: McGraw-Hill, 1966.

Schafer, R. *Aspects of Internalization*. New York: International Universities Press, 1968.

Smith, J. "On the Structural View of Affect." *Journal of the American Psychoanalytic Association* 18 (1970): 539–61.

————. "Rite, Ritual and Defense." *Psychiatry* 46 (1983): 16–30.

Stern, D. "The Early Development of Schemas of Self, of Other, and Various Experiences of 'Self with Other.'" In J. D. Lichtenberg and S. Kaplan, eds., *Reflections on Self-Psychology*. Hillsdale, N.J.: Analytic Press, 1983.

Weber, S. *The Legend of Freud*. Minneapolis: University of Minnesota Press, 1982.

Index

passage to Symbolic order in, 268;
resolution of, xxi
Ontic/ontological distinction, 99
Ontology of personhood, 119–20,
122–23, 126
Ordering principle, 232, 235–36, 249
Origin (human), 227–29, 232,
236–37, 239, 240, 251, 252, 253; in
novel, 254, 257; primal scene as,
255
Original sin, 244–45, 247, 249
Orphanhood, 226, 256
"Other," the, 13, 90, 122, 166,
214–15, 239–40; desire of, 110,
184; different from Freud's "other
scène," 137; dominance of, 89–90;
integration of individual into,
61–63; mediation between subject
and, 164–66
Otherness: excommunication of (*Bleak
House*), 254, 257
Other/other distinction, 11, 90, 99
"Other scène," 137

Paranoia, 114, 132–33
Parapraxis, xii, 14, 15, 185
Parmenides, 152, 154, 156
Paronomasia, 12–13
Pasteur, L., 228n4
Paternal function, 45
Paternal metaphor, 23, 30
Paternal "No," 85, 108
Paternal origin: myth of, 250
Paternity, 186
Patriarchal culture, 235, 251
Paz, Octavio: *Labyrinth of Solitude, The,*
226
Penis: mediator between cut and su-
ture, 174. *See also* Phallus
Perceived, the, 182–83, 184, 185
Perception, 22, 42, 180, 181; distinct
from memory, 182; identity of, 183,
260

Perceptual traces, 37
Perls, F., 216
Phallocentrism, 235–36
Phallus, 83, 168, 176, 186, 252; is/as
lacking signifier, 23–24, 30, 106,
178, 214; as supreme signifier,
109–10
Phenomenology, xv, 40–41, 77
Philosophy, xviii–xix, 156–57, 190,
212–13
Piaget, J., 260n1
Pichon, Edouard, 5n1
Plato, 151, 169
Pleasure principle, 106
Poe, Edgar Allan: "Murders in the
Rue Morgue, The," 254–55; "Pur-
loined Letter, The," 256
Poetry, 204, 273–74
Preconscious, 215, 220
"Pres-ab-sentiality," 144
Presencing, 144, 145–46
Primal scene, 254–55
Primary process, xvii, 8, 152, 195;
words in, xii
Primordial loss, 31
Projective identification, 39, 43–44
Psychical representative, 262–64
Psychic development, xx, 64, 126; in
neonate, 260n1
Psychic energy, xv, 219, 262–66;
transformed into meaning, 81–82
Psychic time, 206–11
Psychoanalysis, 3–5, 19, 64, 139, 152;
addresses failure in oedipal crisis,
268; American, 5–6, 77, 259–75;
and the Being-question, 139–59;
dissolution of ego in, 261; goal of,
215–16; as hermeneutics of desire,
81–82, 83; hermeneutics of unconscious in, 102–11; linguistic interpretation in, 199–200, 201, 203;
models in, xxiv–xv; reductionism
in, 75–77, 80; scientific status for,
113; self liberated in, 77; tem-

Speech, 24, 37*n*8, 141, 216; eroticization of, 42; psychotic, xvii, xxi, 28–29; therapeutic force of, in analysis, xvi, 216–17
Spilka, Mark, 245
Spirit, 107, 134; and death, 100–01
Splitting, 174*n*8, 180; of need and demand, 106. *See also* Subject, split
Statue, idealized, 125, 126
Stoehr, Taylor, 243*n*18, 245
Strachey, James, 173*n*8, 179*n*
Structuralism, xiii, 16, 76, 235
Structural linguistics, 61
Subject, xvii, xxv, 8, 89, 101, 164, 168; authentic, 79; barred, 31, 61–62, 88, 99, 169; becoming, 30–31; Being of, 72; constituted by signifier, 60, 63; of discourse, 202; as emotional force, 136; ex-centric center of, 55–56, 58, 59, 62, 63, 90–91, 274; mediation to ego ideal, 166–67; mediation between Other and, 164–66; objectification of, 9, 10; of psychoanalysis, xxv, 51–74; relationship with signifier, 103–04, 172, 173; relationship of, to symbolic, 72; relationship of, to truth, 190, 212–13; as subordinate to language, 110; term, 163–64; unity of, xvii
Subject, split, 31, 61–62, 88–89, 90, 98–99, 103, 110–11, 210–11; defining, 89–95; Esther in *Bleak House* as, 242–43, 246–47; origin of, 108–09
Subject/image relationship: aggressivity in, 127
Subjectivity, xix, 60, 79, 90–91, 129, 261
Sublimation, xxiii–xxiv, 226*n*2
Substitution (principle), 21, 27
Suicide, 216
Superego, 97
Surrealism, 33
Suture, 177, 180, 184, 187; problem of, 174–77

Suture-cut, 170
Suture of the signifier: relationship with *objet (a)*, 171–78
Swales, Peter J., 51, 53
Symbol, the, 39
Symbol formation, 43
Symbolic, the, xii, xxi, 34, 185
Symbolic equations, 43, 44
Symbolic order, 56, 58, 61, 108, 141, 153, 235, 268; of dream, 70; effected by words, 29–30, 31; Name-of-the-Father ordering principle of, 239; and naming, 149, 150; psychosis and, 21–24, 28, 30; relationship of man to, 140, 141; subject's entrance into, 103–04
Symbolism, 105, 106, 218–19; in Dickens, *Bleak House*, 233, 235, 240–41, 251, 252
Symptoms, 211, 216, 219; structure of metaphor, 4, 203, 204; as trope of movement of unconscious, 211
Synchrony, 61, 185–86
Syntax, 40

"Talking cure," xvii, 33–48. *See also* Analytic cure
Telepathy, 210
Temporality, 72–73, 87–88, 91–95, 98, 99, 102, 107. *See also* Time
Tennyson, Alfred: *In Memoriam*, 229–30
Theme(s), 11–12, 14, 18
Theology, 212–14
Thing-representation, xxi, 215
Third, the, 42, 44
Thomas, Saint, 36*n*7
Thought, 128, 199, 260; identity of, 183; and language, 38–39
Threat, 127–28
Time, 101, 189; relationship of Being to, 143–46. *See also* Temporality
Tol, Herman, 228*n*4
Totality (whole), 97–100, 102
Traces, erasure of, 186, 188